Women, Health and the Family

KT-433-575

Women, Health and the Family

Hilary Graham

Lecturer in Social Policy
University of Bradford

HARVESTER WHEATSHEAF

NEW YORK LONDON TORONTO SYDNEY TOKYO

First published 1984 by
Wheatsheaf Books Ltd
Reprinted by
Harvester Wheatsheaf
66 Wood Lane End, Hemel Hempstead,
Hertfordshire, HP2 4RG
A division of
Simon & Schuster International Group

Printed in Great Britain by
Antony Rowe Ltd, Chippenham, Wiltshire

British Library Cataloguing in Publication Data

Graham, Hilary
  Women, health and the family.
  1. Family—Health and hygiene
  I. Title
  613   RA418.5.F3

ISBN 0-7108-0732-5
ISBN 0-7108-0727-9 Pbk

6   93 92

Contents

List of Figures

List of Tables

Acknowledgements

I would like to record my thanks to the Health Education Council, who provided me with the financial support necessary to write this book. In particular, I would like to thank Ian Sutherland, the Director of Education and Training, and John Harris, the Research Officer until December 1983, for the encouragement they have given me over a number of years.

While the Health Education Council have provided both financial and personal support, I take responsibility for *Women, Health and the Family*. The arguments developed and the views expressed are mine, and not necessarily those of the Council.

I would like to thank the many people, outside the Health Education Council, who have helped me in my search for data on health and the family. They include Jennie Popay, Ioanna Burnell, Ian Cullen, Marion Kerr and Lorna McKee. I am particularly grateful to Ruth Lister and Miriam David for their helpful comments on an earlier draft of the book.

The book, at its various stages, was typed by Sue How. I would like to record my special thanks to her, for her skilful typing and for her moral support over the long writing period.

Beyond my debt to the people I know is my debt to the anonymous women, men and children whose lives are the subject of this book. Over a hundred surveys are recorded in the chapters which follow, representing the experiences of many thousands of families with young children. Without their trust, their help, their time, and above all, their willingness to share their knowledge, this book could not have been written. Without their support, research on family health would end and health professionals and policy makers would know nothing about the reality of family life beyond their own individual experience.

It is therefore to the anonymous families who helped me write this book that I owe my greatest debt.

The author is grateful to the following for permission to reproduce tables and figures in the text: Ioanna Burnell and Jane Wadsworth, formerly of Child Health and Education in the Seventies, University of Bristol for Figure 3.1 and Table 7.3; The Child Poverty Action Group for Tables 6.3 and 6.5; The Family Policy Studies Centre (formerly the Study Commission on the Family) for Table 6.4; HMSO for Figures 3.2 and 3.3; The Journal of Epidemiology and Community Health for Table 5.2; The National Consumer Council for Table 9.5; The National Council for One Parent Families for Figures 2.1 and 2.2; The Office of Population Censuses and Surveys for tables 3.3 and 3.4 and the General Household Survey Unit, OPCS for tables in chapters 3, 4, 6, 7 and 11.

List of Abbreviations

BSSRS	British Society for Social Responsibility in Science
CHES	Child Health and Education in the Seventies
CIS	Counter Information Services
CPRS	Central Policy Review Staff
DHSS	Department of Health and Social Security
EEC	European Economic Community
EOC	Equal Opportunities Commission
GHS	General Household Survey
GP	General Practitioner
NCOPF	National Council for One Parent Families
NHS	National Health Service
OPCS	Office of Population Censuses and Surveys
RCGP	Royal College of General Practitioners
RPI	Retail Price Index
SEG	Socio-Economic Group
SSRC	Social Science Research Council (now the Economic and Social Research Council)

Introduction

This book is about families, and the kind of care they are able to provide for the people who live in them. In most families, care is provided by the woman of the house. A primary concern of the book is therefore with the work that women do for family health.

The book focusses on one particular kind of family: families with children. Families with children are what many people regard as proper families: such phrases as 'starting a family' and 'putting family before career' are used in a way which makes families synonymous with children. Yet, in its focus on parents and children, the book is directed to only a minority of Britain's families. Of the 27 million households in Great Britain in 1981, 7 million (26%) were composed of parents and children. The rest were families containing people living alone, in couples or with others to whom they were not related (DHSS, 1983:a).

While it is important to be reminded that the typical British family is not one with children, statistics on household-type can be deceptive. For although families with children are in the minority, these families accommodate and care for a large proportion of Britain's population. In 1981, the 7 million families with children in Great Britain cared for 26 million people, nearly half the population.

The numerical importance of parents and children in the population has been highlighted by recent social changes which have profoundly affected the lives and living standards of many families with children. These changes have prompted a major debate among health and welfare professionals and among politicians and policy-makers about the role of the family in health. Interest in what families can do and should do to care for themselves 'in sickness and in health' has been fuelled by two factors. It has been fuelled firstly by recent changes in social

1

policy and, more broadly, in public spending on the welfare state. Over the last decade, there has been a marked shift in government thinking in favour of self-help and family care. The present Conservative government, in particular, is firmly committed to increasing the sphere of family responsibility in health care. Professional services have been correspondingly reduced: the number of day-nursery places for children has been cut, for example, as has the number of beds available in old people's homes.

It is not only changes in government policy which have heightened professional and political interest in the quality of health care in the home. A second factor centring around changes within the family has increased concern about the capacity of parents to fulfill the caring roles bestowed upon them. Attention has been drawn to the worsening financial position of many families with children and to the sharp rise in the number of one parent families over the last decade. These two trends — the increase in family poverty and the increase in one parent families — are not unrelated. A significant proportion of poor families are one parent families, and an even larger proportion of one parent families are poor.

Defining and measuring poverty presents many problems, some of which are discussed in Chapter 2. Poverty is defined in this book in terms of household income. Included among the poor are families living on incomes below and up to the current level of supplementary benefit, families living on supplementary benefit and families who have incomes up to 40% above supplementary benefit. Applying this measure to the DHSS data on low income families, we find that families with children now form the largest group among the poor. Through the seventies, it was the elderly who dominated the landscape of poverty: in 1979, men and women over pension age made up over half of those living in poverty. At that time, just over a third (36%) of the poor were parents and children. By 1981, the burden of poverty had shifted sharply. It was no longer the elderly, but parents and children, who predominated among the poor. In 1981, the latest year for which national figures are available, parents and children made up 44% of those in poverty: the proportion of elderly people had correspondingly shrunk to 39% (DHSS, 1983: a). The distribution of poverty in Britain is described in figures 0.1 and 0.2.

Underlying these changes in the distribution of poverty has been a rapid increase in the overall number of people in poverty

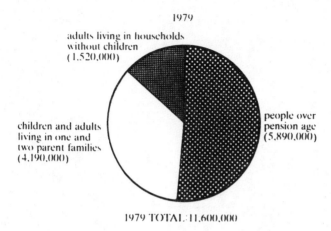

1979

adults living in households
without children
(1,520,000)

children and adults
living in one and
two parent families
(4,190,000)

people over
pension age
(5,890,000)

1979 TOTAL: 11,600,000

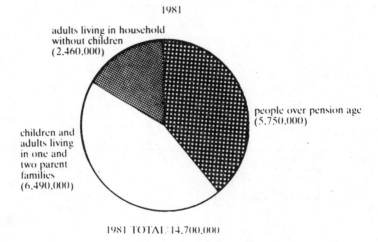

1981

adults living in household
without children
(2,460,000)

children and
adults living
in one and
two parent
families
(6,490,000)

people over pension age
(5,750,000)

1981 TOTAL: 14,700,000

Figure 0.1: People in Poverty, Great Britain, 1979 and 1981
Source: DHSS (1983: a) *Low Income Families, 1981* Tables 1, 2 and 5

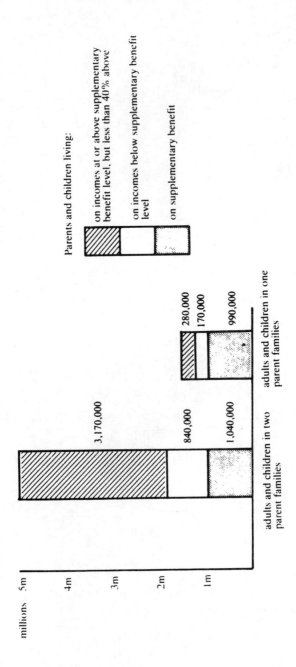

Figure 0.2: One and Two Parent Families in Poverty: Great Britain, 1981
Source: DHSS (1983: a) *Low Income Families, 1981* Tables 1, 2 and 5

since 1979. In that year, 11½ million were estimated to be living in poverty (DHSS, 1983:a). In 1981, the figure was nearly 15 million; a figure including 3½ million children. Accompanying the rise in poverty among parents and children has been an increase in the number of one parent families. The number has more than doubled in twenty years, from under half a million in 1961 to nearly a million in 1981 (NCOPF, 1982). Today, one in seven of Britain's families is headed by a lone parent. Most of these families are headed by a woman, and, according to government figures, over half of one parent families are poor (DHSS, 1983:a).

Living in poverty means living on an income insufficient to purchase the material resources necessary for health. Families in poverty are therefore living in conditions which directly threaten the health of parents and children. The living conditions associated with poverty — poor housing, poor food, inadequate heating and environmental danger — are recognised to have a direct and measurable impact on health. The health of children is seen as particularly vulnerable to such hostile material conditions. The proportion of babies who die around the time of birth is regarded as the most sensitive indicator of child health. This perinatal mortality rate, which measures the proportion of babies who die before, during or within one week of birth, is also regarded as the most sensitive indicator of the welfare of the nation more generally. It sharply — and cruelly — reflects the impact of inadequate resources on the lives of children. The perinatal mortality rate among children born into social class five, where the poorest families are found, is nearly twice that among children in social class one: 17.0 perinatal deaths per 1,000 births in social class 5 compared with 9.7 in social class 1 in 1980. Among illegitimate children, whose mothers are often both poor and alone, the perinatal mortality rate is also high. In 1980, nearly 17 (16.9) babies in every thousand born to unmarried mothers died in the perinatal period: the perinatal mortality rate for legitimate births in that year was 12.8 (MacFarlane & Mugford, 1984).

Shortages have an adverse effect on the health of parents as well as children. Research has highlighted, in particular, the way in which the health of the carer is threatened when money and social support are inadequate. Mothers, who still assume the primary responsibility for caring, are known to be especially vulnerable to illness and stress. The rates of ill-health, physical and mental, are thus high among working-class women who care for young children.

At a macro-level, these relationships are widely recognised. We read frequently of the continuing class inequalities in child health, and the risks of depression among housebound mothers. Yet, we know very little about how the social environment of working-class families threatens the health of children born into them. We know very little either about why the material and human resources available to parents provide less protection against mental stress to mothers than fathers, and offer less support for working-class mothers than for middle-class mothers. While the family is at the centre of the debate about health and welfare, the question of how the family manages its health remains unasked.

It is this question which is raised here. The chapters which follow attempt to provide some answers by drawing together the material which illuminates the hidden world of family care. They are concerned with health care in a literal sense: with the care that promotes health. The book considers how the basic necessities — money, housing, fuel, food and transport — are distributed between and within families. It describes, too, the human resources necessary for health. It looks at the way in which women (and some men) organise their day to combine successfully the myriad roles that lie behind the deceptively simple label 'mother'. It looks at the roles they perform as cook, cleaner and childminder, as health teacher and public relations officer and, most importantly, as the housekeeper whose job it is to ensure that the family stays both healthy and solvent.

'Health care' is rarely a term used to describe what mothers do for the family. Instead, we tend to restrict the term to the work of paid professionals: doctors, nurses, midwives and health visitors are the people we more readily identify as members of the health care team. It is this professional health service we have in mind when we make assessments about the quality of health care in Britain. And when politicians speak of crisis, it is to a crisis in the professional health service that they refer. It is in the context of the National Health Service that the crisis of demand is discussed, a crisis fanned by the needs of Britain's increasingly aged population. It is in this context, too, that commentators describe the crisis of cash, noting that reductions in the capital and human resources invested in health care will result in shortages in beds and equipment and in chronic understaffing.

By comparison, we hear little about the crisis in the informal and unpaid health service. Any recurrent crises of cash that it may face go unrecorded: so, too, do its shortages of equipment and staff. While the public costs of health care, borne by taxation, are very much publicised, the private costs of care remain private. Yet, it is this informal sector which provides most of the care. The direct involvement of professionals, by comparison, is very small. Most children are cared for in their families: over 99%. Most of the elderly, over 95%, too, live in the community. Even among groups like disabled children and the frail elderly who are recognised to be in need of constant nursing, the family provides the front-line care.

The extensive and intensive care provided by the family forms the basis on which the professional services have evolved. Professional health workers, like doctors and health visitors, do not provide an alternative to the family: rather they have a range of skills which they employ in order to improve the quality of care that families provide. Doctors diagnose and prescribe treatments for the patients who come to them: they do not nurse the sick. Similarly, health visitors listen and advise: it is left to mothers to put their advice into practice.

The consequence of this obvious but fundamental division of labour is that professional health workers tend to see, and to deal with, only the tip of the iceberg. Dealing only with the tip, it is easy for professionals and policy makers to lose sight of the other health service and to equate health care with the care they provide. This tendency is reflected in the terms we use to describe health and welfare. We talk about GPs and health visitors providing a *primary* (not a backup) health care team; we talk of them seeing patients and not fellow health workers and visiting clients and not carers.

Once people are defined as patients and clients, it is difficult to see them as the producers as well as the consumers of health services. This problem is avoided in some of the categories favoured in recent policy documents. These talk of parents, families and communities, terms which themselves convey the commitment and obligation we have to care for one another. However, like the more established labels of patient and client, these newer concepts blinker our ways of seeing health care in another respect. The terms are all gender-neutral. They cover both men and women and they tell us nothing about the sex of the carer, or the cared-for. Yet gender is a crucial dimension of health care. Women form the majority of patients in the National

Health Service: women visit their GPs significantly more often than men, and there are significantly more women than men among the disabled and in psychiatric and geriatric hospitals. Women, too, form the majority of health workers, paid and unpaid. Within the welfare state, the vast majority of nurses, midwives, health visitors and auxiliary staff are women: most social workers are women too. Within the home, the majority of mothers are wage-earners, going out to work along with the fathers. But this sharing of income-production has not been associated with a concomitant sharing of health responsibilities. Mothers remain the primary carers in two parent families. In one parent families, too, we find women carrying the burden of health care. For while some fathers are lone parents, the majority (over 85%) of one parent families are headed by women. It is mothers, therefore, who have the task of marshalling the resources their families need for health.

In exploring how mothers go about this task, the book focusses on families where the vital health resources are likely to be in short supply. It focusses on poor families and one parent families. In poor families, income and the material assets that money buys, are insufficient for health. One parent families face not only material scarcity; they can face a shortage of parent-power as well. These two groups of families are not mutually exclusive, but each experiences, in an extreme way, many of the resource problems that beset all families. Poor families and one parent families do not, however, only highlight the specific problems mothers face in working for family health. They highlight, too, many of the general processes which govern the organisation of women's health work. In particular, poverty and single parent-hood highlight the impact of two aspects of Britain's social structure which have a major influence on health care in the home: class divisions and gender divisions. Family poverty reflects the impact of the class structure on parents bringing up young families. Poor parents are parents who, disadvantaged within the labour market, find themselves restricted to low-paying jobs or to unemployment. Single parenthood reflects the impact of gender divisions on family health. Because women are the primary carers, it is mothers who typically take responsibility for the children when a marriage ends. This division of re-sponsibility not only affects women's work in the home: it also seriously limits their employment opportunities in the labour market. Women's employment has traditionally been limited to jobs where pay and security are low. Their low pay reduces the income of many two parent families, keeping them on the margins of poverty. However, it is Britain's one parent families who experience the full impact of women's disadvantaged position in the labour market. The poverty of one parent families is recognised to be a direct result of these disadvantages.

In placing particular emphasis on the class structure and the sex role system, other important aspects of our social structure are obscured. Yet, these aspects also affect what mothers are able to do for their families' health. Eclipsed, for example, is the question of racial divisions and area of residence. But race and area of residence are known to influence a family's access to key health resources: to secure employment, adequate housing, safe play areas, efficient transport and good quality medical services. Further, race and area of residence are known to combine with other structures of disadvantage. One parent families, for example, are not only predominantly working-class and female-headed. Many one parent families are black and more still find themselves confined to the poorest areas of our inner cities. While not ignoring them, this book does not give these structures the same prominence as it accords to social class and gender divisions.

The book is selective in other ways too. Firstly, because of the attention paid to one parent families, the chapters devote less space to other families in poverty. They make little reference, for example, to family size, and the poverty of large families. They make little reference either to families caring for disabled children or to families in which the parents are themselves incapacitated. However, in outlining the problems faced by families where money is short and the staff are over-stretched, the chapters describe the lives of many parents coping with extra children or with the burden of disability. For, to a considerable extent, the problems experienced by such parents are the same as those of other families — but on a larger and more daunting scale.

The book is selective in a second respect. It is concerned with how families organise themselves to protect the health of those they care for. It is therefore primarily interested in the routine of family life and not with families during times of transition. It does not describe the process by which single parent families are formed: by women becoming mothers alone, by marriage breakdown or by death. Similarly, it does not describe the process by which two parent families are created: through cohabitation, through marriage and remarriage. Research into the constitution and reconstitution of families is reviewed elsewhere (Hart, 1976; MacIntyre, 1977; O'Brien, 1982; Burgoyne and Clark, 1983). So, too, is the literature on the psychological effects on parents and children of marriage breakdown (Wallerstein and Berlin Kelly, 1980; Richards and Dyson, 1982). The chapters focus instead on the relatively long periods in the lives of one and two parent families where health work is organised according to established routines, rather than the times of change when these everyday arrangements are abandoned.

Thirdly, as noted earlier, the book is concerned with health care, not with medical care. This is not only a semantic distinction; it reflects its orientation to what families, rather than professionals, do to safeguard health. Nonetheless, professional care plays an important part in family health, and the utilisation of medical services cannot be divorced from a family's health experiences. The evidence on utilisation is included in Chapter 3 and the question of access to medical services is raised again in Chapters 9 and 11. However, medical care is not treated as a separate resource for family health in the way that income, housing and food are. This is partly because the design and delivery of professional health care has been a recent focus of research and is extensively reviewed elsewhere (Blaxter, 1981; Elbourne, 1981; RCGP, 1982; Townsend and Davidson, 1982). Including such a large and complex issue within the brief of this book would have reduced the already limited space that can be devoted to other, less widely-publicised areas of family health. More particularly, the decision to include the informal family services, even at the expense of the formal services of the Welfare State, reflects the book's dominant concern with those health resources which are secured through the work of parents. It is this question, of how families work for health, that is explored in the chapters which follow.

The book is divided into five parts. Parts I and II describe the patterns of family life and family health in Britain. Part I is concerned with *Understanding Family Life*, and examines the position of parents and children in the 1980s. Chapter 1 considers the concept of the family and describes the diversity of living situations encompassed within it. Chapter 2 looks at the concept of poverty and its implications for our understanding of family health. The chapter examines, too, the concept of single parenthood, and identifies some of the differences which exist between and within one and two parent families.

Part II describes the *Patterns of Family Health* in Britain. It focusses on social class and sexual divisions, and maps out the impact of these aspects of our social structure on health. Chapter 3 discusses the question of social class and health, examining the class differences in health and the utilisation of professional health care among parents and children. Chapters 4 and 5 are concerned with the impact of gender divisions on family health. This issue raises two connected, but distinct, questions concerning the relation between gender and health-work on the one hand, and gender and health on the other. Chapter 4 considers the way in which gender shapes the kind of work that parents do for their families. It looks at women's contribution to family health within the home and at the contribution they make through their paid work outside the home. This chapter also looks at the role that women play in the health policies of prevention and community care which, at first glance at least, seem to involve us all. Chapter 5 considers the relation between gender and health. It reviews the evidence on the health-effects of caring, concluding that health work has its own occupational hazards. It reviews, too, the evidence on the health of women and children in female-headed one parent families, comparing their health experiences with those found among the more typical and traditional two parent households.

Parts I and II outline the structures of family life and family health within which parents work. Parts III and IV describe what this health work involves: the resources it consumes and the responsibilities it entails. Part III examines the *Resources for Family Health*, noting how these resources are shared out between and within families. Chapter 6 examines the question of family income, and Chapter 7 describes the quality of housing available to families. Chapter 8 discusses the family diet. While nutrition plays a vital role in health, it is in this area that women most commonly make savings when money is short. Chapter 9 examines the provision of transport, an issue not usually included in discussions of family health, yet one which influences women's access to the health-promoting services they need for the family. A recurrent theme in these four chapters concerns the internal division of resources within the family. While most families have sufficient resources to safeguard health, these resources are not necessarily distributed in line with respon-

sibilities. Mothers may thus find themselves responsible for
feeding the family, but without an income sufficient to meet their
nutritional needs. They may assume the task of buying food and
escorting their children to the doctor, but not have access to the
family car.

While Part III considers the division of family resources, Part
IV turns to the division of the *Responsibilities for Family
Health*. It identifies a number of important tasks that women
perform in their role as mothers: meeting basic needs, nursing the
sick, teaching about health and mediating with professionals. In
addition, it identifies coping with crisis as an activity which
underlies these various dimensions of women's health work. As
in the professional world of the NHS, crisis-management appears
an enduring feature of successful caring.

The evidence presented in the first four parts of the book
describes how families, in different circumstances, cope with
their responsibilities for health. It describes, in particular, how
mothers work to keep their families going. Such work, it suggests,
involves both 'health keeping' and 'housekeeping'. Mothers must
ensure not only physical survival, but financial survival as well.
Where money is tight, the two roles can conflict. In order to keep
the family solvent, mothers on low incomes cut back on the
resources necessary to keep them healthy: food, fuel and clothes.
Such compromises are not equally borne by all members of the
household. Typically, the needs of some family members are
sacrificed in order to meet the needs of others: the diet of the
children is protected at the cost of that of the parents, fuel is
conserved during the day to have the house warm for the
returning breadwinner. Not infrequently, the burden of sacrifices
falls heavily on the mother: her commitment to the welfare of her
partner and her children can involve her in reneging on her
commitment to look after herself.

These complex patterns of compromise and sacrifice illuminate how families with children meet their current health
responsibilities. However, the evidence presented in this book
has a wider relevance. It can provide a much-needed insight into
the reality of family care, at a time when the social context of
family care is changing rapidly. Looking at families with children
now can help us appreciate what these changes in family life and
family policy mean for health and for the lives of women in the
future.

It is this focus on future patterns and policy that Part V

provides. It looks at the concept of choice, central to recent initiatives in the field of health, in the context in which mothers work for health. It highlights the crucial issue which policy-makers and professionals have to confront as they design and deliver new health policies in the 1980s: can families take on more responsibility, with less state support than they currently receive and still keep together and keep healthy?

The book directs our attention to this critical issue by asking the obvious but neglected question of how families cope with the responsibilities they have.

A NOTE ON THE TEXT

Comments and quotations drawn from government reports and empirical studies of family life have been included to illustrate the main text of the book. This material can be read on its own, or alongside the main text which it is designed to illuminate.

Part I
UNDERSTANDING FAMILY LIFE

1 Defining Families

1.1 THE FAMILY IN GOVERNMENT POLICY

Most people grow up in families. For most of us, it is families which met our health needs in childhood: for warmth and shelter, for love and comfort. Families, too, serve as our first and most significant health teachers. In adulthood, most people create new families (often more than once) to support them 'in sickness and in health'. In old age, it is our family, again, who cares most and does most for us.

The importance of the family in health care has been underlined by the changes described in the Introduction. Changes in family life and changes in social policy have sharpened public awareness about what families can and should do for their dependents. However, in much of the debate about family responsibility, the family has remained undefined. It features, instead, as a kind of catch-all category which embraces those forms of care which the state does not (or should not) provide.

When discussing the position of the elderly and handicapped, policy makers generally invoke a wide concept of the family unit (DHSS, 1981:a; DHSS, 1981:b). It is seen as a kinship network spanning three or more generations, and involving relatives who do not necessarily live in the same household.

The concept of the family takes on a more precise meaning when children are the subject of policy. Here, the family is typically regarded as a two-generation structure, marked out by the lines of responsibility which run between parents and child-(ren). Over the last decade a series of government reports have stressed the obligation, and to a lesser extent the right, that parents have to provide basic health care for themselves and their children. A theme of the 1976 Court Report on the Child Health Services, for example, was the need for professionals to share

17

rather than deliver health education and health care. More recently, Court's emphasis on developing a partnership between parents and professionals has been subsumed within a wider economic strategy on health and welfare. Health policy in the 1980s is concerned with shifting rather than sharing responsibilities for health care. The emphasis today is less on what professionals can do for families, and more on what families, supported by voluntary efforts in the community, can do for themselves.

the importance of the family must be reflected in the organisation and delivery of health services for children ... [Professionals] should see themselves as partners with parents: prepared and willing to give them explanation and advice about their children's health[1]

A prime objective (in child health care) should be to encourage the development of self-help and community activities involving children, and through these to help parents look after children better. Both organised voluntary effort and informal care (from family, friends and neighbours) play a vital role in the network of community based support.[2]

The question of definition is not the only problem, however, with 'the family'. Whether their objective is partnership, as proposed by the Court Report, or self-help, as advocated by *Care in Action*, health policies not only presume an appreciation of what the family is. They presume, also, an understanding of what families do. In particular, they presume an understanding of how families work to promote and protect the health of their members. An appreciation of the health work of families, however, has been slow to develop. The Court Report noted in 1976 that an effective child health service, sensitive to the responsibilities and rights of parents, requires 'an understanding of the child's family circumstances' (Court Report, 1976:170). Four years later, the Central Policy Review Staff, in its report on *People and Their Families*, again recorded the need for a greater political and professional awareness of family circumstances. Today the same theme is still being stressed. In the series of reports issued by the Study Commission on the Family, we are reminded that we still know too little and assume too much about parents and children.

the advantages and disadvantages which children experience are to a large degree those of their parents, both in material terms and in the standard of care that they provide. It is in this context that provision for children must be seen.[3]

Services will never reflect the importance of the family for health, education and welfare until there is a clear understanding of the diversity of family patterns of which lone parenthood is but one element.[4]

The fact that policy makers and professionals lack what the Court Report calls 'an understanding of the child's family circumstances' might not be a problem if all British families conformed to a standard shape and size. The concept of the family, although unspecified, would have a precise meaning, reflecting the current patterns of child-bearing and child-rearing in the community. The problem is that this homogeneity does not exist. There is no such thing as 'the family' in the sense of one accepted model of family life. Instead, variety is the norm. Only one quarter of British households contain children. A smaller proportion still are households with a male breadwinner, a non-employed wife and dependent children. Among the economically active population, only 5% are married men with two dependent children and a wife not in paid work (Coussins and Coote 1981:9).

1.2   DEFINING FAMILIES

Faced with the variety of family forms, statisticians prefer to talk of 'households' rather than 'families'. Households are groups of individuals who live at the same address and share their living accommodation. This may sound a rather minimal way to characterise family life but it provides the baseline for the collection of data. It provides, too, a baseline for this book, which is concerned with one particular group of households: households in which a parent or parents live with their dependent children. It is in this specific sense that the term 'family' is used here. In this book:

A family is a household in which a man and a woman live alone or together with their dependent child(ren) sharing a common system of housekeeping.

From this minimal definition, we can identify the kind of activities necessary to sustain a shared address and a common system of housekeeping. Maintaining a family involves the parent or parents in two sets of activities: income production and housework/childcare. To sustain a household, parents must generate an income sufficient to meet the family's needs. They need to find the money for housing, heating, clothes and food for themselves and their children. To maintain the household, they must also meet the social responsibilities of family life: organising their time to ensure that meals are cooked and clothes washed, that the house is clean and safe, and their children are cared for. In most households, these tasks constitute two full-time jobs: income production and housework/childcare. Each involves at least eight hours a day of time and energy. Where there are two parents, both are thus fully occupied in keeping the family going. However, recent changes in employment have complicated the organisation of these family responsibilities.

Looking at the position of two parent families, we find, firstly, that an increasing number require more than one full-time worker to meet their financial obligations. In such circumstances, the purchasing power of the family can only be protected by cutting the person power available in the house. In families with two wage-earners, there is particular pressure on those who shoulder the main responsibility for housework and childcare. They carry the double burden of paid and unpaid work.

Secondly, while more parents need to work to keep two parent families out of poverty, a growing number of parents are unemployed. Unemployment haunts adults in low-paid jobs. It is thus families already enduring the ill-effects of low pay who are most likely to suffer the poverty of unemployment. The DHSS cohort study of unemployed men found that, among men with children, one third were already living in poverty before they lost their jobs (Millar, 1983). Unemployment leads to a further deterioration in family income and living standards, with families becoming poorer the longer the parents have been out of work. As income falls, so does the investment that parents can make in protecting the health of their children. A study based on data from the Family Expenditure Survey found that families enduring long-term unemployment were able to spend little on children's clothes and shoes. The average amount spent by the long-term unemployed on children's shoes in the course of a year was just over £2.00, well below the price of one new pair of shoes (Bradshaw, Cooke and Godfrey, 1983).

Such figures starkly illustrate the effects of unemployment on family health. These ill-effects might be tempered, however partially, if unemployed fathers invested their energies in housework and childcare. However, research suggests that this transfer of effort from income-production to family care does not occur on a large scale. In families in which the father is unemployed, as among families in which both parents work, women continue to be responsible for the home and the children (McKee, 1983).

Turning to the position of one parent families, we find that the trade-offs between income production and health care are more complex. For here the labour of two must be performed by one. In the attempt to cope with the demands of income-production, housekeeping and childcare, many single parents surrender their role as wage earner. Nearly half of all one-parent families rely on the state for their main source of income, releasing energies for the full-time task of caring for their children. However, like in many two-parent families, the solutions are not always adequate for the problem: low income and understaffing are chronic features of an increasing number of British families. Nonetheless, it is an obvious but important point that when talking about families — two parent families, one parent families, employed families and unemployed families — we are talking about households which have managed to survive these problems. We are talking about units of parents and children who, whatever the difficulties, have remained together in their own homes.

1.3 IDENTIFYING DIFFERENT TYPES OF FAMILIES

Maintaining a household — a shared address and a common system of housekeeping — involves parents in a range of responsibilities. As we have seen, parents need to provide material resources — money and the goods that it buys. They need to provide, too, the human resources of time and energy necessary to keep themselves and their children in health. The material and human resources available to parents are closely related to the family's economic circumstances (principally income) and its social structure (the number of parents it contains). These two dimensions — economic circumstances and social structure — provide a framework in which we can identify different types of families.

It enables us to identify families according to their financial circumstances; to distinguish between families who live in poverty and those with incomes sufficient to keep parents and children above the poverty line. It allows us to identify families according to their household structure; in particular, to identify whether there are one or two parents responsible for the maintenance of the household.

The two dimensions provide an indicator of the purchasing power and person power of families. Where the income-generating capacity of a household is high, both money and time are released for spending on health: as, for example, in families where one or more parents are in highly-paid jobs. Where this capacity is low, the financial and human investment which parents can make in family health is likely to be severely restricted. This is most likely to be the case in families where the parents are limited to low paying jobs and in families where there is only one potential wage earner.

It is important to note that economic circumstances and household structure serve as indicators only. These variables influence the pattern of resources within the family: they do not determine it. The presence of two parents does not guarantee better care for the children. In fact, marital breakdown can enable the remaining parent to devote more resources, both material and emotional, to the children (Marsden, 1973:62; Weiss 1979 Chapter 4; Pahl 1980:328). Similarly the presence of a high wage earner does not ensure a high standard of living for all the family. Money can be distributed in such a way that there is 'poverty amidst plenty'. One parent may be well provided for, while the spouse and children go short.

One compensation for being a single parent is that there is opportunity to be closer to the children. There is no second adult in the household with whom parenthood must be shared, to whom loyalty is owed, who distracts the parent's attention and discourages the development of separate understandings with the children.[5]

The existence of poverty amidst plenty highlights an important point. In talking about the impact of economic circumstances and household structure on family health, we must be careful to distinguish between households and individuals. These two dimensions can help us identify *households* which are likely to be under-resourced. But they alone do not determine, and cannot reveal, the quality of life of *individuals* within these households. Individual well-being is shaped by the distribution, as well as the volume, of resources in the family. An appreciation of the division of resources and responsibilities is central to this book and the issue is explored in detail in Parts III and IV.

NOTES

1. Report of the Committee on Child Health Services (1976) *Fit for the Future*, Cmnd. 6684, Vol.1, pp.85-6 (The Court Report).
2. DHSS (1981: a) *Care in Action*, pp.37 and 46.
3. Central Policy Review Staff (1980) *People and their Families*, HMSO, p.12.
4. Popay, J., Rimmer, L. & Rossiter, C. (1983) *One Parent Families: Parents, Children and Public Policy*, Study Commission on the Family, p.52.
5. Weiss, R (1979) *Going It Alone*.

2 Diversity and Inequality in Family Life

2.1 CHILDREN AND THEIR FAMILIES

There are twelve million children under sixteen in Great Britain (National Report, 1981 Census). They presently constitute about a quarter of the population but by the end of the century this is likely to have fallen slightly (CPRS 1980:9). The available data on children is not without its limitations, as other researchers have noted (ibid.). A serious weakness is the absence of up to date statistics on family health, at a time when the economic position of parents and children is known to be deteriorating. Because there is typically a two year time-lag between the collection and publication of social data, we have to wait until 1986 before we have detailed figures on family life in 1984.

Despite these problems, general patterns are clear. The vast majority of children live in families. Over 99% of Britain's children live with one or both of their parents. Under 1% are in the care of local authorities. Even here, the family plays a major role. Half of the children in care are in residential homes run by local authorities or by voluntary organisations. The remainder live in families: with their parent(s), guardians or, increasingly, with foster parents (CPRS 1980:16).

Although most children grow up in families, their experience of family life is far from uniform. Chapter 1 identified household income and household structure as two major determinants of childhood experience. This chapter defines these two dimensions more exactly.

The two sections below consider the question of family poverty and the definition of a one and two parent family. The fourth section provides some demographic information about the situation of one parent families in Britain, while the final section adds

24

a word of caution about the interpretation of such statistics on family life.

In 1981: 99% of Britain's children lived in families.[1]
  34% of these children (3½ million) lived in or on the margins of poverty.[2]
  14% of families in Britain were one parent families.[3]
  55% of one parent families lived in or on the margins of poverty.[2]

Sources: 1. CPRS, 1980;   2. DHSS, 1983: a;   3. NCOPF, 1983.

2.2   FAMILIES IN AND OUT OF POVERTY

Since the nineteenth-century investigations of Seebohm Rowntree, poverty has been defined by governments in terms of a precisely-defined level of household income. Rowntree calculated the income necessary for physical survival, acknowledging that his calculations deliberately ignored the fact that family life involved more than 'bare subsistence'. Despite these reservations, Rowntree's calculations served to mark the boundary between poverty and welfare in William Beveridge's plans for the post-war social security system. The level of supplementary benefit was designed to keep those dependent on it out of poverty. It represented the poverty line. Similarly, today, the rates of supplementary benefit are taken as the poverty line for households of different size and structure. From November 1983 to November 1984, the supplementary benefit rate (excluding housing costs) for a family with two parents and two children under 11 is £61.80 a week.

My primary poverty line ... was a standard of bare *subsistence* rather than living ... The dietary I selected was more economical and less attractive than was given paupers in workhouses. I purposely selected such a dietary so that no-one could possibly accuse me of placing my subsistence level too high. All other necessary household expenditure was calculated after careful investigation on a similarly economical basis ... A family living upon the scale allowed for in this estimate ... must never go into the country unless they walk ... They must write no letters to absent children, for they cannot afford to pay the postage. They must never contribute anything to their church or chapel, or give any help to a neighbour which costs them money ... Nothing must be bought but what is absolutely necessary for the maintenance of physical health and what is bought must be of the plainest and most economical description.[1]

Measuring poverty in terms of household income implies that poverty has an objective status. Yet, while the experience of poverty is real enough, as a concept it is ambiguous and value-laden. What counts as a minimum income reflects the prevailing standards of living in the community. What a particular family needs is determined by the standard of housing, diet, dress and social activity to which other families have access. The 'poverty line' represents a political decision about the distribution of wealth: it indicates 'the community's view about what standard of living is the minimum to be tolerated in a society as wealthy as ours' (Marsden 1973:3).

It is not sufficient to assess poverty by absolute standards; nowadays it must be judged on relative criteria by comparison with the standards of living of other groups in the community ... beneficiaries must have an income which enables them to participate in the life of the community.[2]

Poverty is an inability to achieve a standard of living allowing for self-respect, the respect of others and for full participation in society. In the last analysis, to be poor is not just to be located at the tail end of some distribution of income, but to be placed in a particular relationship of inferiority to the wider society. Poverty involves a particular sort of powerlessness, an inability to control the circumstances of one's life in the face of more powerful groups in society.[3]

The fact that poverty is culturally defined does not prevent it having objective effects. One of the most clear-cut results of poverty is ill-health. The empirical relationship between poverty and ill-health is well-documented and is explored in Chapter 3 (3.4 and 3.5) and Chapter 5 (5.5). What is less widely appreciated is that ill-health is implied in the definition of poverty. Poverty, as we have seen, is a level of income incompatible with health. Being out of poverty, therefore, means enjoying a standard of living which, however marginally, sustains the health of oneself and one's family. Being on the poverty line means living on an income which, in theory at least, is sufficient to protect health. Being in poverty means having an income which is incompatible with health.

The link between poverty and health is closer and more complex still. For evidence suggests that the poverty line represented by supplementary benefit is set too low to sustain good health. A variety of studies confirm that the minimum income necessary for health is significantly above the current rate of supplementary benefit for adults and children (Burghes 1980; Piachaud 1979; Piachaud 1981). The rates of supplementary benefit payable to children have been found to be most out of line with needs. David Piachaud concludes from his study of the cost of keeping children in health, that the rates are well below the minimum needed (Piachaud, 1981:14). The stringency of the supplementary benefit rates has led researchers to broaden the band of poverty. Included among the poor are those whose incomes are up to 40% above the level of supplementary benefit. They are typically identified as being 'on the margins of poverty'. Official recognition that the 40% level provides a more realistic measure of poverty is underlined by the fact that the Department of Health and Social Security uses this measure in its calculation of *Low Income Families* (DHSS, 1983:a).

It is this broader and more comprehensive measure of poverty that is adopted here. Although not without limitations, it provides the best available indicator of the economic circumstances of Britain's families. With it, we can identify two types of family: those in and those out of poverty. In this book:

A family in poverty is one whose needs exceed the financial resouces available to meet them. Their total income falls below or up to 40% above the level of supplementary benefit.

A family out of poverty is one in which the household income is sufficient to meet the needs of parents and children. Their income is more than 40% above the level of supplementary benefit.

Over the last twenty years the proportion of the population in poverty according to this definition has increased substantially. In 1960, 14% lived in poverty (Townsend, 1981: 67). In 1979, the proportion was 22%; by 1981, it was 28%, nearly 15 million people (DHSS, 1983: a). Among the poor are a significant number who live on supplementary benefit, the base line of poverty. In 1981, nearly 5 million of Britain's 15 million poor were dependent on supplementary benefit for their survival. The figure for 1983 was 7 million, one in eight of Britain's population (figure released by Anthony Newton to the House of Commons, 27 April 1983).

Some groups in the population are more vulnerable to poverty than others: the old, the young, the handicapped and those in large families. In the 1970s, the elderly formed the largest group in poverty (Layard, Piachaud and Stewart, 1978). Since then, however, the burden of poverty has shifted from the elderly on to children and their families. By 1981, families with children were the largest single group living in poverty (DHSS, 1983:a).

The economic recession of recent years has brought with it a disturbing increase in the number of families living in poverty or on its margins. Whereas the elderly dominated the landscape of poverty during the 1960s, the current decade has witnessed an increasing incidence of low incomes among families with children.[4]

A large and growing group of families in poverty are families headed by a lone parent. It is to this second dimension of family life — namely, household structure — that the chapter now turns.

2.3 ONE AND TWO PARENT FAMILIES: DEFINITIONS

In 1974, the government inquiry into the circumstances of one parent families published its report. The *Report of the Committee on One Parent Families*, the Finer Report, defined a one parent family as 'a father or mother living without a spouse (or not cohabiting), with his or her never-married dependent child or children aged either below 16 or 16-19 and undergoing full-time education'. This definition explicitly excludes families with cohabiting adults; it excludes too, families in which the children are no longer dependent. From our point of view, Finer's is a useful definition by virtue of what it implies about the care of children. Finer's concept suggests that *a one parent family is a particular kind of household with children whose organisation rests on the work of one parent*. By extension, a lone parent is someone who has daily responsibility for the maintenance of the home and the care of the children. This definition is close to that adopted by Townsend in his survey of poverty (Townsend, 1979). It is similar, too, to the terms employed by the Commission of European Communities, in their survey of poverty in the EEC (Friis, Lauritsen & Steen 1982). They identified lone parents as those who have 'de facto the sole responsibility financially and educationally for the child/children' (ibid.: 2). This definition does not specify the sex of the lone parent, just that they are coping alone. In fact, the majority of single parents are women: most data on lone parents are therefore data on women who are bringing up children on their own.

The standard definition of a one parent family, as a household of one adult with one or more dependent children, is not without problems, however. Not all one parent families are households in this sense. In fact, this definition is known only to cover about half of one parent families. This is partly because it excludes one parent families with dependent children aged 16 or over. More importantly, it is a definition which excludes one parent families living in a household with other adults (Redfern, 1982:23). It is estimated that nearly half of Britain's one parent families share their homes, often with their parents. Because of this pattern of multi-occupation, the 1981 household census is not regarded as a reliable guide to the numbers of one parent families. For this reason, estimates are usually derived from an analysis of Child Benefit order books. These estimates suggest there are about one million single parent families caring for over 1.6 million children (Popay, Rimmer & Rossiter 1983:9).

The one million lone parents are something of a self-selected group. They are mothers and fathers who, when faced with an illegitimate birth, a marriage breakdown or a bereavement, find they can manage on their own. In focussing on functioning households, we necessarily lose sight of those who are over-whelmed by the financial and domestic burdens. We lose sight of the many single parents who, when confronted with the pressures of coping alone, enter new relationships. And we lose sight of those whose children are taken into care. A large proportion of children in local authority care are from one parent families. This proportion is estimated to be over 50% (NCOPF, 1980: 5). Data on one parent families are data on the survivors; they are likely to underestimate the gravity of the problems facing those who try to bring up children on their own.

On the basis of our definition of a one parent family, we can also define a two parent family. *A two parent family is a particular kind of household with children whose organisation rests on the work of two parents.* In such a household, the daily responsibility for income-generation and the maintenance of the home and the care of the children is shared between two parents. This definition does not specify how the responsibility is divided: it tells us only that there are two parents whose labours, potentially at least, can help keep the family going. In fact, because of the traditional division of tasks between parents, it is mothers who take responsibility for the day-to-day care of the children and upkeep of the home (Land, 1981). Having primary responsibility for the children is therefore not unique to lone parents: it is a condition shared by most married women as well. While their responsibilities are similar, the context in which they meet them is different. Single parents work always alone.

I think one of the hardest things is being entirely responsible for everything, on your own, in a situation where normally things are shared. I mean being responsible for earning a living, raising children, everything, and never even getting a break. It is very hard.[5]

The majority of families are two parent families. According to latest estimates, the figure is 86% (NCOPF 1982: 19). While still a minority, the proportion of one parent families has increased sharply over the last two decades. In the twenty years from 1961 to 1981, the number of one parent families more than doubled (Figure 2.1). These statistics, however, mask important differences within the two groups of families, as we see in the next section.

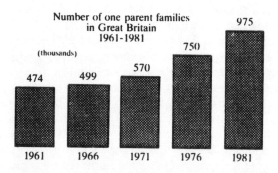

Number of one parent families
in Great Britain
1961-1981
(thousands)

Figure 2.1: Number of One Parent Families in Great Britain, 1961-81
Source: National Council for One Parent Families (1983) *One Parent Families*, p. 19

2.4 ONE AND TWO PARENT FAMILIES: SOME CHARACTERISTICS

One and two parent families are not homogenous and distinct groups. Reflecting the changing patterns of marriage and divorce, parents and children move in and out of one parent families over time.

Among two parent families, most children live with their natural parents. But an increasing number live in reconstituted families, with a natural parent and a step-parent (CPRS 1980: 17). In some respects, these step-children appear to be more disadvantaged than children in one parent families (Burnell and Wadsworth, 1981; Popay, Rimmer and Rossiter, 1983: 33-4).

Step-children may well represent a new, but less visible, 'at risk' group in the child population. Their vulnerability underlines the fact that having two parents does not guarantee material and emotional security in childhood, any more than having one parent threatens it.

One parent families represent an even wider diversity of living situations. As Figure 2.2 indicates, it is a term which covers a wide range of experiences. While inadequate, it is generally considered preferable to other, more pejorative, labels. Classifications which distinguish 'normal families' from 'one-parent families', 'intact households' from 'broken homes' betray a negative orientation which characterises popular attitudes to single parents (Popay, Rimmer and Rossiter, 1983: 18-25).

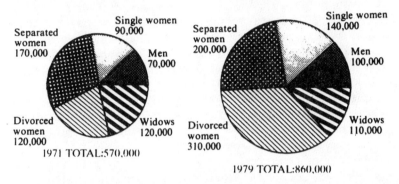

Figure 2.2: Number of One Parent Families by Marital Status: Great Britain, 1971 and 1979

Source: National Council for One Parent Families (1983) *One Parent Families*, p. 19

The most significant divisions within the single parent group are those of sex, marital status and race. As Figure 2.2 indicates, the majority of one parent families are female-headed. Eight out of nine lone parents (88%) are lone mothers (NCOPF, 1982: 19). A similar proportion of one parent families in the United States is composed of unpartnered women with children (Nielsen and Endo, 1983: 131). Most single parents in Britain were once married, with marriage breakdown and not death being the major cause of lone parenthood (Figure 2.2).

These divisions of sex and marital status are reflected in family income. In general, lone fathers and widowed mothers are financially better off than single, separated and divorced mothers. The higher incomes among lone fathers are due to the fact that most lone fathers are able to continue earning after separation; the higher income of widows reflects the relatively generous way in which Britain's social security system has treated them as compared to other groups of lone mothers.

Ethnic differences are also known to exist among one parent families. National data, however, are not available to measure the extent and the effects of these differences. Evidence indicates that white and West Indian women are more likely to become single parents than mothers from South Asian and Chinese communities in Britain (Ballard, 1982; Barrow, 1982; Jackson, 1982). In the United States, the impact of race on family structure and family income has been more systematically investigated. National data record the fact that a higher percentage of black than white families are female headed and poor. In 1971, one in three black families was female headed, and one half of these families were below the poverty line. Among white families, one in ten was female-headed, and one quarter of lone white mothers were bringing up their children in poverty (United States Commission on Civil Rights, 1974).

Reflecting the importance of sex and racial differences in income, one parent families are concentrated in the poorest areas of Britain. In particular, they are disproportionately represented in inner-city areas. Data from the 1981 census suggests that while 14% of all families nationally are headed by a single parent, in the inner-city areas of our conurbations the figure is much higher. In Manchester, for example, the figure is 27%: the highest figure found outside London. However, within London, the proportion of one parent families rises to nearly one third in some London boroughs. In Lambeth, Hackney, Hammersmith, City of London and Camden, over 30% of families are single parent families (Table 2.1).

Data from the 1981 census have been used to measure the quality of life enjoyed in these inner city areas of Britain. The Department of the Environment's Inner City Directorate, for example, has drawn a national map of urban deprivation from the 1981 census. Significantly, as in other analyses, the proportion of one parent families is identified as an indicator of urban disadvantage (Redfern, 1982). The Directorate notes that one parent families, like ethnic minority families and pensioners, are concentrated in areas with the worst amenities and the poorest opportunities. As a result, the distribution of social deprivation closely matches that of one parent families. Outside

London, social deprivation was found to be at its worst in Manchester. Within London, too, single parents are concentrated in areas of greatest need. Among the London boroughs, Lambeth, Hackney, Hammersmith and Camden are among the worst ten identified by the Directorate. These areas are characterised by poor housing, overcrowding, unemployment and high mortality rates (Inner Cities Directorate, 1983).

Table 2.1: Single Parent Families in London: Percentage of Families with Children Headed by Lone Parents, 1981

London boroughs	%
Bexley	9·9
Brent	21·2
Bromley	11·9
Camden	30·0
City of London	30·7
Ealing	16·2
Hackney	32·0
Hammersmith	31·1
Harringay	22·2
Harrow	11·4
Islington	28·9
Kensington and Chelsea	27·3
Lambeth	33·2

Source: National Council for One Parent Families (1982) *One Parent Families 1982*, p. 19.

2.5   CONCLUSION: THE NEED FOR A DYNAMIC PERSPECTIVE

To understand the changing patterns of family life, we need to take a dynamic view of childrearing. However, much of the data are cross-sectional. They provide snapshots of family structure and income level at particular points in time. Yet we know that parents (and children) move in and out of marriages and in and out of poverty. While only a minority of children are cared for by a lone parent at any one time, many more have experienced or will experience life in a one parent family before they reach their sixteenth birthday. It is estimated that one marriage in three now ends in divorce, with the result that one in five of today's children are likely to live through the break-up of their parents' marriage (Haskey, 1983). This figure does not include those children who are born to unmarried mothers or those who become part of a single parent family as the result of a parent's death.

The importance of a dynamic perspective on single parenthood is underlined by recent historical research. This suggests that single parenthood, far from being a modern phenomenon, has been a feature of British society at least since the industrial revolution. One parent families, it seems, were very much part of Victorian family life. Michael Anderson has demonstrated that illegitimate birth rates are little, if at all, higher than in the mid-nineteenth century (Anderson, 1983: a: 4). Looking at figures on marital breakup, through divorce and death, he notes, too, that the rates for the early and late nineteenth century are very similar to those of today:

> During the 1970s well over one million dependent children were affected by the divorce of their parents. But the Victorians, too, had problems of marital disruption and of single parent families. We do not know how many marriages were broken by divorce or separation in the past ... What we do know is that, of couples who married at the average age in the 1860s, around one in three had their marriage broken by death within 20 years. This figure is remarkably close to the death-plus-divorce expectations of couples marrying today. The chances that a child would experience a broken home were higher right up to the end of the nineteenth century than they were during the 1970s. Broken families on our present scale are not new.[6]

The need for a dynamic perspective on childhood is equally important if we are to understand the impact of poverty. While the experience of lone parenthood can be short-lived, the experience of poverty is more enduring. The arrival of children places a strain on the finances of many families. Children are born into working-class households when, with the mother out of paid employment, family incomes are at their lowest. Since the family's financial circumstances typically improve only when the mother and later the children themselves join the labour market, the experience of childhood for many is one of chronic poverty. However, the rise of unemployment threatens this economic upturn in the life-cycle of many working-class families. With high youth unemployment, reaching 50% among Britain's eighteen-year olds in 1983, the poverty of childhood can endure into adulthood.

Longitudinal studies of child health and development help correct the static pictures of family life presented in national statistics. Major longitudinal studies were conducted at twelve-year intervals from 1946. From the 1970 study, we know that under half of the children born to unsupported women in 1970 were in one parent families five years later (Burnell and Wadsworth, 1981). We know, too, from this survey that these children had been joined by others whose married parents had split up. Such studies are a rich source of data: however, the CHES study, as the last national cohort study, is already fourteen years old. Its children were born in 1970, before the recent increase in divorce and remarriage and the sharp rise in unemployment and family poverty.

In addition to the lack of longitudinal data on children born in the 1980s, there have been recent cut-backs in national data-collection (Macfarlane and Armstrong, 1983). Data on the numbers dependent on supplementary benefit, for example, are no longer prepared annually. They are released every other year: thus, figures on poverty in 1981 were released in 1983, while 1985 figures will not be available until 1987.

The shortage of data, from both independent longitudinal surveys and from government figures, is likely to act as a fetter on our understanding of family health in the future.

NOTES

1. Rowntree, B.S. (1941) *Poverty and Progress*, pp.28 and 34.
2. DHSS Parliamentary Under-Secretary, House of Commons, 6 November 1979.
3. Kincaid, J. (1973) *Poverty and Inequality in Britain*, p.159.
4. McNay, M. & Pond, C. (1980) *Low Pay and Family Poverty*, Study Commission on the Family, p.1.
5. Itzin, C. (1980) *Splitting Up*, p.60.
6. Anderson, M. (1983: b) 'How much has the family changed?', *New Society*, Vol.66, 1093: 143.

Part II
PATTERNS OF FAMILY HEALTH

3 Social Class and Family Health

3.1 INTRODUCTION

A person's health is closely related to his or her position in society. Personal health is known to vary between rich and poor, between black and white and between men and women. Of these features of our social structure, social class has been the most extensively investigated. It is working-class families, and working-class children, who have been found to suffer most from illness, disability and premature death. Moreover, most families are working-class, and one parent families are disproportionately represented in working-class communities.

The evidence on class differences in health has been summarised in a series of influential reports. There are the three national longitudinal studies of child health begun in 1946, 1958 and 1970. In addition, there have been a number of government working parties and committees concerned with health inequalities: the Court Report on the Child Health Services (1976), the Merrison Report on the National Health Service (1979), the Short Report on Perinatal and Neonatal Mortality (1980) and the Black Report on Inequalities in Health (1980). Finally, and most recently, there is the joint research on deprivation and disadvantage sponsored by the Department of Health and Social Security and the Social Science Research Council. While addressing a broader brief, this research, too, has provided both detailed reviews and new evidence on the relationship between social class and health (Blaxter, 1981; Blaxter and Patterson, 1982; Brown and Madge, 1982: Madge, 1983).

These reports and enquiries provide a rich source of data on class inequality and health. This chapter does not aim to summarise their findings but only to pick out certain recurrent themes in the literature. It discussed four areas: the measurement of social class, the position of one and two parent families in the class structure, the link between social class and child health and finally, the link between social class and adult health.

Of these areas, it is the nature of the link between social class and health that is most controversial. Controversy turns on the question of cause and effect: is personal health a cause or a consequence of social position? The Black Report on Health Inequalities, for example, points to the way in which health reflects, and is shaped by, social position. In other words, it argues that health is primarily determined by social structure (Townsend and Davidson, 1982: 122-3). The DHSS/SSRC research into deprivation and disadvantage similarly places emphasis on the material differences between individuals and families in explaining patterns of health (Blaxter, 1981). This chapter, too, favours a perspective which identifies the distribution of material resources as a crucial determinant of health.

While the balance of scientific opinion currently identifies social class, and social structure more generally, as the causal variable in health, a minority of studies suggest a very different model (Illsley, 1955). They argue that cause and effect may be wrongly identified: it may be health which determines social position and not social position which determines health (Stern, 1983). The evidence to support this theory comes from the data on social mobility within the class structure. Given Britain's high rates of social mobility, it is possible that those in poor health drift down the class structure, producing artificially high rates of morbidity and mortality among adults in social classes four and five.

In highlighting the problems of causal inference, this theory points to some of the limitations of the materialist perspective. However, it is not generally accepted as an alternative capable of explaining more than a small part of the association between health and wealth. Nonetheless, the existence of such conflicting models should not be forgotten in the chapters which follow.

3.2   THE CONCEPT OF SOCIAL CLASS

According to official surveys, about half Britain's children (and their parents) are classified as working-class. What is meant by social class in these surveys? How is it measured? How does its definition and measurement structure our understanding of the relation between social class and family health?

Social class is the central concept in the study of health and family life. It is employed as a measure of the social and economic differences within society and the impact of these differences upon individual expectations and experiences. Occupation is generally thought to be the best available measure of social and economic inequality and one, moreover, which reflects the structured nature of inequality. The social class classification of occupations most frequently employed in British surveys is the Registrar General's classification, developed by the Office of Population Censuses and Surveys (OPCS). This is based on a six-fold classification of occupation, with three non-manual groups (social classes 1, 2 and 3NM) and three manual groups (social classes 3M, 4 and 5). The division between non-manual and manual occupations marks the line between the two major social classes: the middle class and the working class.

While the Registrar General's social class classification is used in the Census, a slightly different classification of occupation is used in the General Household Survey. This annual national sample survey of about 10,000 households is a major source of data for Parts II and III of the book. In the General Household Survey, occupations are allocated to one of eighteen categories, known as socio-economic groups. The socio-economic groups, in

Table 3.1: The Social Class of Some Occupations in the Registrar General's Classification

	Social Class	Occupations Included
I	Professional etc.	accountant, clergyman, doctor, lawyer
II	Intermediate	teacher, farmer, manager
III NM	Skilled Non-Manual	secretary, shop assistant, sales representative
III M	Skilled Manual	bus driver, electrician, miner (underground), cook
IV	Partly Skilled	agricultural worker, bus conductor, machine sewer, packer, telephone operator
V	Unskilled	laundry worker, office cleaner, labourer

turn, are grouped together to form seven larger categories: professional; employers and managers; intermediate non-manual; junior non-manual; skilled manual; semi-skilled manual and personal service; and unskilled manual. These larger Socio-economic Groups roughly correspond to the Registrar General's classification, but they are not identical. Like the Registrar General's social classes, the General Household Survey's Socio-economic Groups provide us with a measure of the way in which an individual's position in the labour market shapes their health, income and living standards. In this sense, they both provide a measure of the impact of social class on family health and family resources.

In assigning individuals to a social class or a Socio-economic Group, their sex and their position in the household are often crucial. Men are generally assigned according to their own occupation. Women and children are generally classified according to the occupation of their husband or father. Husbands and fathers thus earn their social class directly, through their job: other household members have their social class ascribed indirectly, through their relation with the class-bearing man. Thus, when we talk of 'working-class men', 'working-class women' and 'working class children' we are not using categories that are equivalent. Working-class men are men in manual occupations: working-class women are women fathered by, married to or living with men in manual occupations. Working-class children, similarly, are children living with a man with a manual job. Only when the woman lives alone is the ascription 'working-class' likely to describe her occupational status.

The anomalous position of women and children complicates the task of interpreting class data on health. For example, it is well documented that working-class women are particularly vulnerable to illness, but because the statistics on women's health refer to men's occupational status it is difficult to discover the contribution that women's employment histories make to their physical and mental health. Among children, the risks of accidental death are closely linked to social class (Figure 3.2). The differences are unlikely to spring from the work fathers do, but from the physical environment their income secures. However, class statistics on child health do not directly tap the environment of childhood.

Social class and health are linked ... The factors which contribute to this link are all part of our 'standard of living'. Housing conditions, poor nutrition, occupational and environmental hazards and unhealthy habits are almost inextricably mixed just because they are so class related, and very rarely are researchers given the chance to disentangle them.[1]

The Registrar General's method of measuring social class has been criticised on a number of grounds (Nicholls, 1979; Nissel, 1980). Three assumptions, in particular, have been challenged. Firstly, in classifying families according to the occupation of the head of household, the system assumes that all members share the same social class and this social class is reflected in the present, or last, occupation of its head. This assumption has a number of questionable implications. It implies that the occupation and earnings of other household members do not significantly affect the family's overall socio-economic position. Conversely, it implies that loss of earnings through the unemployment of other wage-earners does not alter the social class of the family. It implies further that all household members share the same standard of living as the household head. Family resources are assumed to be pooled and equitably shared to ensure that no one is in poverty while others live in affluence.

Secondly, the Registrar-General's classification assumes that occupation is the best indicator of social class. It is based on occupational criteria rather than on income or education or housing indicators which may provide a more accurate measure of an individual's social situation. This has particular implications for the economically inactive: for housewives, children, the elderly and the disabled. For the quality of their lifestyle is more directly linked to the physical environment of the private domain: to the quality of housing and play-space, to the facilities in the community and to the level of such public services as medical care, schools and transport.

Thirdly, the Registrar-General's system rests on a particular hierarchy of occupations. While based on the pecking order traditionally associated with men's jobs (in which non-manual is ranked higher than manual, and clerical skills above technical skills), it is assumed also to be one suited to identifying the social class ranking of female occupations. It can thus be used to identify the social class position of female-headed households. However, the structure of women's employment differs from men's. Most women work in non-manual ('middle-class') jobs, but their job security and rates of pay are significantly worse than those found in many male manual trades (EOC 1983).

Fourthly, because the Registrar General's classification is a classification of occupation, families with no one in a job must be incorporated in other ways if they are not to become classless. Typically, they are classified according to the last occupation of the head of household. However, such a solution obscures the fact that such families are economically dependent not on the labour market, as the source of earnings, but on the state, as the source of benefits. Again, this raises particular problems for the classification of women and their children. Most lone mothers rely on supplementary benefit for their financial survival: it is their relationship with the state and not with the labour market which determines their economic position.

Taking these limitations together, commentators have concluded that the occupation of the head of household, while indicative of the economic standing of the father, is not a reliable guide to the social position and health experiences of his dependents. In female-headed households, the Registrar-General's classification loses even this restricted validity. As a result, other indicators of social and economic status have been designed to overcome these problems. The Social Index, constructed by Osborn and Morris (1979) for the 1970 British Births and CHES (The Child Health and Education in the Seventies) Surveys, is expressly designed for the economically inactive who rely most on the immediate material and social environment of their family and neighbourhood.

The Social Index is composed of seven socio-economic variables, relating to occupational status, education and housing situation (see below). These seven variables, like those incorporated into the Registrar General's classification, are measures of social and economic inequality. However, they are ones which relate specifically to the home and cultural milieu of the child.

Items Comprising the Social Index

Classification of father's occupation (Registrar General's
    classification, 1970)
Parent's education
Social rating of neighbourhood
Tenure
Crowding index (persons per room ratio)
Bathroom availability
Type of accommodation

Source: Osborn, A. & Morris, T. (1979) 'The rationale for a
composite index of social class and its evaluation', *British
Journal of Sociology*, 30, 1: 48

In broad outline, the Social Index and the Registrar General's
classification paint a similar picture of the social structure.
Families who fare badly on the Social Index emerge as social
class five in the Registrar General's schema. Families who are
rated as advantaged on the Social Index are heavily concentrated
in social classes one and two. However, the Social Index is a more
sensitive and discriminating measure of childhood disadvantage.
Firstly, as a composite score, the Social Index directly taps the
child's physical and social environment. Secondly, it offers a
measure of social stratification for families in which there is no
father or occupation to provide the basis of the classification.
Thirdly, as a result of these two features, it can identify social
disadvantage within the social classes. While concentrated at the
bottom of the class structure, disadvantage is found in families
across the Registrar General's classification. Only families in
social class one escape. Using the Social Index it is thus possible
to identify groups of disadvantaged familes — like one parent
families — who are lost within the traditional tiers of the class
system.

3.3 THE SOCIAL CLASS OF BRITAIN'S FAMILIES

Data from the 1981 census on the class background of Britain's
children suggest that most children still live in households headed
by a parent whose present or last occupation was a manual one.
Regional differences, as in other areas of family life, are pronounced. These differences are revealed in Table 3.2. The table
indicates that 23% of children in West Yorkshire live in social
classes one and two; in Buckinghamshire the proportion is 40%.
Conversely, while 57% of West Yorkshire's children live in
manual working-class households, 42% of Buckinghamshire
children are from working-class homes.

  The proportion of working-class families has been shrinking
throughout the century. The reasons for this shift in Britain's class
structure are complex. However, it is clear that it has not been
associated with a major redistribution of wealth from rich to
poor. The shrinking proportion of working-class families does
not reflect so much the increasing number of families achieving

Table 3.2: Social Class of Children Under 16 by Economic Position
of Head of Household (10% sample)

*Social class of
economically active
heads of household*

| | Children under 16: | | | |
| | W. Yorkshire | | Buckinghamshire | |
	No.	%	No.	%
1	1,917	4	1,285	9
2	9,011	19	4,350	31
3 NM	4,101	9	1,231	9
3 M	16,242	35	4,064	29
4	7,349	16	1,412	10
5	2,683	6	390	3
Armed forces	1,177	3	475	3
Inactive heads	4,174	9	818	6
	46,654	100	14,025	100

Source: OPCS (1982) *Census 1981 County Report, West Yorkshire
    Part 2*, Table 49 and *Census 1981 County Report, Bucking-
    hamshire Part 2*, Table 49.

middle-class incomes and life-styles as the contracting number of
working-class jobs. During the 1960s and 1970s, the number of
jobs available to unskilled and semi-skilled workers shrank by
almost half: from nearly five million to two-and-a-half million.
The decline is still continuing.

In 1921, 14% of male employees were in non-manual
occupations,[1]
    in 1951 the figure was 20%,[1]
    in 1971 it was 31%,[1]
    in 1981 it was 45%.[2]

Sources: 1: Royal Commission on the Distribution of Income &
    Wealth;
    2: approximate figure only, calculated from OPCS (1982)
    Census 1981 County Reports.

The decline in unskilled and semi-skilled employment has
fuelled divisions in the labour market. In particular, it has fuelled
divisions between those whose jobs offer them secure and rising
life-time earnings and those whose working life is spent in low-

paid jobs and unemployment. This division between 'primary' and 'secondary' employment provides the backcloth to the class differences in living standards. It also provides the backcloth to sex differences in employment and earnings. The concept of a 'dual labour market' is introduced again in Chapters 4 and 6.

Most two-parent families are working-class: and so, too, are the majority of single-parent families. In part, this reflects the class distribution of Britain as a whole; in part, it reflects the greater risks of single parenthood which face working-class mothers and fathers. Available evidence suggests that working-class children are more likely to experience life in a one-parent family than are middle-class children. Using data from the 1958 National Child Development Study, Ferri (1976) found that the proportion of children not living with both parents was lowest in social classes one and two (one child in eighteen) and highest in social class five (one child in seven). This finding is supported by Burnell and Wadsworth (1981) in their analysis of one and two parent families in the 1975 CHES study. They found that a greater proportion of five year olds living in one parent families had fathers in social class five. It appears that the material conditions of family life in working-class communities, as Chapters 6 to 9 record, offer less protection to marriages than those found in middle-class households.

Burnell and Wadsworth noted that one parent families are more likely to come from working-class communities; they also found that children in one parent families were more likely to move down the social scale than children in two parent families. Having only one parent increases the likelihood that a child will end up in social class four or five and thus in a position of social disadvantage. Using the Social Index (described in section 3.2), Burnell and Wadsworth compared the situation of five-year-old children in different types of family. Their results, reproduced in Figure 3.1, highlight the social and economic disadvantages faced by one parent families. Twice as many children living with one parent at the age of five were found to be disadvantaged compared with those in two parent families (60% compared with 26%). The use of the Social Index highlighted differences within, as well as between, family types. Figure 3.1 underlines the importance of the sex of the lone parent in determining the social and economic position of the children.

Although only approximate measures, both the Registrar General's classification and the Social Index point to wide social

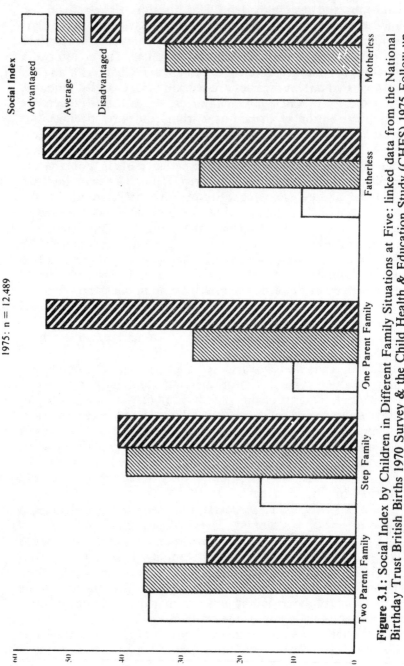

Figure 3.1: Social Index by Children in Different Family Situations at Five: linked data from the National Birthday Trust British Births 1970 Survey & the Child Health & Education Study (CHES) 1975 Follow-up

Source: Burnell, I. and Wadsworth, J. *Children in One Parent Families,* University of Bristol, Figure 7.1

and economic differences among Britain's families. The class differences are reflected most clearly in the health experiences of middle- and working-class families. These health experiences are mapped out in the two sections below. Differences in the economic position of one and two parent families are also associated with health differences: these are discussed in Chapter 5.

3.4 SOCIAL CLASS AND CHILD HEALTH

Children still die in our lifetime for nineteenth century reasons.[2]

The relationship between social class and health is at its closest in childhood. The statistics on perinatal and infant mortality are regarded as the most sensitive indicator of the nation's health. They provide disturbing evidence of the way in which health is related to the class background of the family into which the child is born (see Table 3.3). In 1931, children born into social class five were twice as likely to die in the first year of life as their brothers and sisters in social class one. By 1951, the infant mortality rate had halved. But the class ratio was unchanged. By 1971, the infant mortality rate had fallen again, but the class ratio had widened to 2.5:1. Clearly, class inequalities in child health are not diminishing over time.

Stillbirths:	foetal deaths after 28 completed weeks of gestation
Perinatal mortality:	stillbirths and deaths in the first week of life
Neonatal mortality:	deaths in the first 28 days of life
Post-neonatal mortality:	deaths at ages over 28 days and under one year
Infant mortality:	deaths at all ages under 1 year

Concern with the class differences in infant mortality has focussed on the perinatal period. Policy-makers and health professionals have directed their attention to the medical facilities available during pregnancy and childbirth and in the early weeks after birth. Class inequalities, however, are sharpest in the post-neonatal period, between twenty-eight days and one year

Table 3.3: Stillbirth and Mortality Rates in the First Year of Life for Legitimate Births by Social Class, 1979

Social Class		Rate			
	Still-birth*	Peri-natal mortality*	Neo-natal mortality†	Post-neonatal mortality†	Infant mortality†
1	5·2	10·3	6·5	3·3	9·8
2	6·3	11·8	6·9	2·8	9·7
3 NM	6·8	12·7	7·2	2·6	9·8
3 M	8·1	14·3	7·5	3·9	11·4
4	9·3	16·5	9·1	5·2	14·3
5	9·6	18·7	10·7	8·1	18·7
All	7·7	13·9	7·7	3·9	11·6

* per thousand live and stillbirths
† per thousand live births

Source: Office of Population Censuses & Surveys (1982) *Mortality Statistics 1978, 1979: Perinatal & Infant (Social and biological factors)*, Series DH3 No 7, HMSO, Tables 6-10.

Table 3.4: Stillbirth and Mortality Rates in the First Year of Life by Country of Birth of Mother, 1979

Country of birth of mother	Stillbirth rate*	Perinatal mortality rate*	Neonatal mortality rate†	Post-neonatal mortality rate†	Infant mortality rate†
All countries	8·0	14·6	8·2	4·5	12·6
United Kingdom	7·7	14·3	8·0	4·4	12·5
Irish Republic	8·6	15·1	8·0	3·4	11·4
Australia, Canada and New Zealand	5·6	8·8	4·4	4·4	8·8
New Commonwealth					
India and Bangladesh	12·0	20·2	10·1	4·9	15·0
African Common-wealth	10·3	18·5	10·4	3·3	13·6
West Indies	11·1	17·7	8·9	4·5	13·5
Pakistan	11·8	21·4	11·7	8·0	19·7

* per thousand live and still births
† per thousand live births

Source: Office of Population Censuses and Surveys (1982) *Mortality Statistics 1978, 1979: Perinatal & infant (social and biological factors)*, Series DH3 No 7, HMSO, Tables 20-24.

after birth. As Table 3.3 records, three times as many babies in social class five die in the post-neonatal period as in social class one. It is at this time that, outside the protected environment of womb and hospital, the baby confronts for the first time the material conditions of the home. A similar pattern appears when race and not social class is the indicator of disadvantage. Analyses by mother's country of birth reveals the children of mothers born in the New Commonwealth and Pakistan have rates above those of children whose mothers were born in the United Kingdom. Again, the differences are more marked in the post-neonatal period, than in the periods before, during and immediately after birth (see Table 3.4).

It was apparently true that it was as safe in the 1930s to have a baby at home without antenatal care and without specialists to call upon, provided one came from social class 1, as it was to have a baby from a social class 5 background twenty years later. This simple example underlines the tremendous quantitative importance of social factors in relation to the health and deaths of children.[3]

A review of the state of health of the people of the different groups suggests that, as income increases, disease and death-rate decrease, children grow more quickly, adult stature is greater and general health and physique improve.[4]

Environmental factors have long been recognised as major determinants of the class differences in child health (McKeown, 1979). It is the poor material environment of working-class children which is seen to be responsible for their poorer health and greater vulnerability to premature death. The causes of childhood death showing the strongest class gradient are those which are environmental in origin — reflecting the child's exposure to poor housing, poor nutrition and unsafe play areas. The evidence on childhood mortality is summarised in Figure 3.2. Accidents, perhaps the most direct measure of environmental danger, are the largest single cause of childhood deaths. They alone account for 30% of all deaths in childhood. They also show the sharpest class gradient (see Figure 3.2). Road traffic accidents account for over half the fatal accidents to children between the ages of one and fourteen. However, among pre-school children, most fatal accidents happen in the home (Macfarlane and Fox, 1978): it is the over-fives who are the main victims of death on the road. Infections, parasitic and respiratory diseases, the other traditional environmental killers of children, show a similar, but less pronounced, class gradient. Together, these diseases account for 20% of all childhood deaths. The

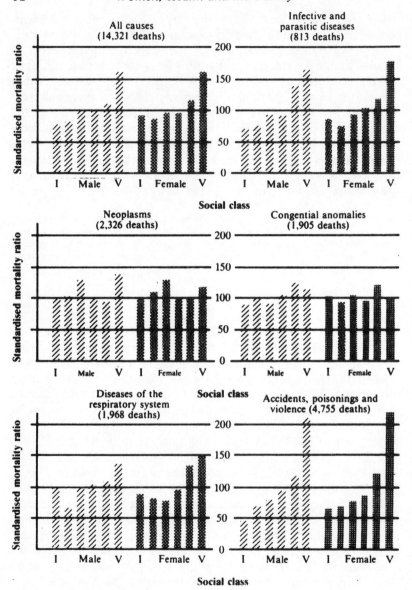

Figure 3.2: Social Class and Mortality in Childhood: Males and
          Females, 0-14.

Source: OPCS (1978) *Occupational Mortality 1970-72, Decennial Supplement, England
         and Wales,* Series DS No 1, HMSO, Figure 7.4. Crown Copyright;
         reproduced with permission of the Controller of HMSO.

remaining major causes of death in childhood — cancer and congenital anomalies — have no marked class gradient.

Turning from mortality to morbidity, class differences are still apparent. However, the class gradient is less clear and less consistent across the range of data on childhood illness. The longitudinal studies of childhood show a consistent class gradient on many indicators of physical development and health (Spence, et al, 1954; Davie, Butler and Goldstein, 1972). Working-class children experience more illness, particularly respiratory and infectious diseases (bronchitis, mumps, whooping cough, pneumonia). Interestingly, these differences found in the detailed longitudinal surveys of childhood are not replicated in the General Household Survey. This relies on self-reported illness. In the case of children, researchers are tapping mothers' perceptions of their children's health, perceptions influenced by their own class position. GHS data suggest no consistent class trend for children as a whole.

Childhood mortality statistics and the morbidity data from the longitudinal studies record the impact of social class on child health. Reflecting this impact, we would expect working-class children to make proportionately more use of the health service than middle-class children. However, this matching of 'use' to 'need' is not apparent. Although the data are limited, and often contradictory, they indicate that there is an Inverse Care Law in operation (Tudor Hart, 1971). Those in most need of the professional services make least use of them. The Inverse Care Law is particularly in evidence in the take-up of preventative services: the use of dental and child health services and the rates of immunisation are lower among working-class children (Townsend and Davidson, 1982:81-84; Blaxter, 1981:156-67).

In explaining the higher rates of mortality and morbidity among working-class children, and the lower take-up of professional services, considerable attention has been paid to the behaviour of the mother. The Newcastle 1000 Families study, for example, introduced the concepts of 'deprivation' and 'deficiency' as measures of the standard of parental care, while the 1946 national longitudinal study of child health assessed 'maternal efficiency' on the basis of data collected by health visitors. More recently, in the DHSS/SSRC study of deprivation and disadvantage, the role of mothers in transmitting childhood illness has been reviewed again. However, like the 1946 survey, the researchers concluded that the determinants of both health and health behaviour lay in the material and social environment of the home (Douglas and Bloomfield, 1958; Blaxter and Paterson, 1982). The deprivations and deficiencies belonged not to the mother, but to the society in which she worked to secure health for her family.

The findings of such surveys shed some interesting light on the operation of the Inverse Care Law. They raise the possibility that the non-utilisation of community health and GP services may reflect not so much a failing on the part of mothers as their superior knowledge of the constraints of family life. Seen in this context, what initially appears as inefficiency to an outsider, emerges as the most sensible use of the mother's time, energy and money. Where money is short, the costs and benefits of any action must be carefully weighed. Where the costs, however marginally, outweigh the benefits, a mother cannot always afford to take advantage of health services for herself and her family. Even with a National Health Service which is free at the time of use, the indirect costs can be prohibitive. This complex and little-explored area of family decision-making is opened up in Part III and IV.

As far as costs are concerned, there are several reasons why the costs of using a free service will be greater for working class users from the lower S.E.G.S. than for those from the higher ones. Time spent travelling will be greater because they are more reliant upon public transport ... Also, they are likely to have further to travel, for the areas in which they live are poorly endowed with medical facilities. The costs of waiting are likely to be higher, since they cannot so easily make appointments by telephone.[5]

3.5 SOCIAL CLASS AND ADULT HEALTH

In adulthood, as in childhood, social class is associated with differences in individual health. Health statistics reflect the contrasting life-styles of rich and poor in Britain: the different living and working conditions found in the home, the labour market and the local community.

The impact of these conditions is felt most directly in the mortality statistics. As in childhood, death from accidents and respiratory diseases show steep class gradients. So, too, do the so-called diseases of affluence (the malignant neoplasms and diseases of the circulatory system identified in Figure 3.3). As Figure 3.3 indicates, cancer and heart disease should be more aptly named diseases of poverty.

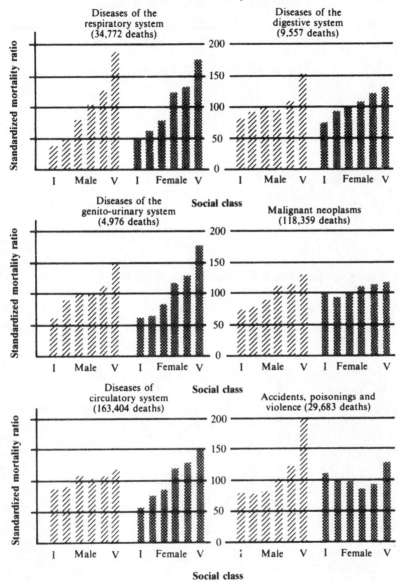

Figure 3.3: Social Class and Mortality in Adulthood (Men and Married Women, 15-64)

Source: OPCS (1978) *Occupational Mortality 1970-72, Decennial Supplement, England and Wales,* Series DS No 1, HMSO, Figure 4.4. Crown Copyright; reproduced with permission of the Controller of HMSO.

Table 3.5: Social Class and Morbidity: Persons Reporting a Limiting Long-Standing Illness, Great Britain, 1980

	% reporting limiting long-standing illness	
Socio-economic Group	Males — all ages	Females — all ages
Professional	12	13
Employers & managers	14	15
Intermediate & junior non-manual	17	18
Skilled manual	18	18
Semi-skilled manual and personal service	20	25
Unskilled manual	24	28
	(Number in sample = 14,879)	(Number in sample = 16,016)

Source: General Household Survey 1980 (1982) Table 7.8, p. 137.

Table 3.6: Social Class and Doctor Consultations: Average Number of GP (NHS) Consultations Per Person Per Year, Great Britain, 1980

Socio-economic Group	Males — all ages	Females — all ages
Professional	2·9	4·1
Employers & managers	3·5	4·4
Intermediate & junior non-manual	3·7	4·6
Skilled manual	3·7	4·9
Semi-skilled manual and personal service	4·0	5·4
Unskilled manual	4·3	5·5
	(Number in sample = 14,928)	(Number in sample = 16,074)

Source: General Household Survey 1980 (1982) Table 7.16, p. 141.

Reflecting the class influences on mortality, the rates of morbidity and medical consultation are also class related. Tables 3.5 and 3.6 summarise the data from the General Household Survey on chronic illness and GP consultations. Table 3.5 indicates that twice as many men and women in unskilled manual households as in professional households suffer from a chronic illness which limits the performance of their everyday activities: a statistic in line with the class differences in mortality. The pattern of GP consultations (Table 3.6) appears less closely related to social class. While men and women in the lowest socio-economic group consult their doctor more frequently, the differences are not as pronounced as the mortality and morbidity statistics would suggest. The level of consultation among working-class families does appear to match their need. An Inverse Care Law is in evidence again.

The patterns of health and health-care in adulthood reveal not only social class differences, but sex differences as well. Figure 3.3 demonstrates the higher rates of male mortality. The greater vulnerability of men to premature death would suggest that they would have more ill-health and more medical consultations than women. However, it is women who are more likely to report periods of chronic ill-health (see Table 3.5). It is women, too, who record the greater use of their GP (see Table 3.6).

These sex differences suggest that social class is not the only dimension of our social structure with a determining influence on health. Chapters 4 and 5 explore the influence of a second major feature of our society, namely the division between the social worlds of men and women.

NOTES

1. Bedale, C. & Fletcher, T. (1982) *The Times Health Supplement*, 12th February, p.15.
2. *Report of the Committee on Child Health Services* (1976) 'Fit for the Future', Vol. 1, Cmnd. 6684 (The Court Report), p.6.
3. Royal College of General Practitioners (1982) *Healthier Children — Thinking Prevention*, p.1.
4. Boyd Orr, J. (1937) *Food, Health and Income*, p.55.
5. Le Grand, J. (1982) *The Strategy of Inequality*, p.32.

4 Gender Divisions and Family Health:

Women's Work for the Family

4.1 INTRODUCTION TO CHAPTERS 4 AND 5

Social class is not the only dimension of social structure to have a pervasive impact on individual health. How much individuals get in terms of the material and human resources which determine health is also influenced by their race, sex and regional background. Reflecting these differences in access to resources, data suggest that there are racial, sexual and regional inequalities in health (Brown and Madge, 1982:111-14).

Here, the focus is upon one of these areas of inequality. Chapters 4 and 5 examine the impact of sex inequalities on family health, introducing issues to be explored in later chapters. The question of sex and gender is singled out for discussion because, like social class, it relates directly to the organisation of family life. Social class influences the distribution of resources *between* families: the distribution of income and housing for example. The influence of sexual divisions is more complex. Assumptions about the needs and obligations of men and women play a primary role in shaping the distribution of resources *within* families: both between the sexes and between the generations. However, their effects are not restricted to the domestic domain. In the labour market, too, there are sex differences in employment and earnings. With the increasing numbers of female-headed families, these differences have become an important factor in fuelling inequalities *between* families.

The patterns of resource allocation within and between families are seen to reflect a structure of sexual divisions as deep-

58

rooted and pervasive as the class divisions traditionally associated with Western societies. This structure is linked to family health in obvious and important ways.

Firstly, there is the link between sexual divisions and the organisation of work, both within and beyond the family. Most parents, whether living alone or with a partner, work hard to promote the health of their families. Mothers and fathers, however, rarely do the same kind of work. By custom, if not by choice, men are responsible for securing the family income while women are responsible for maintaining the home and rearing the children. Women who, either alone or with their partner, attempt to break down these traditional sex roles by taking responsibility for earning the family income find themselves in a labour market which similarly differentiates between 'men's work' and 'women's work'. Moreover, women's work typically carries with it less security, less prospects and less pay.

Chapter 4 explores the question of women's work for the family. It looks at women's domestic work and the contribution that women make to the health of their partners and their children. This is the subject of section 4.2 below. The chapter also examines the world of paid employment and the relation between women's caring role in the home and their position in the labour market. The implications of women's low pay for family health are discussed in section 4.3. Finally, the chapter considers the way in which women's work is represented in social policy. Because women are the caretakers of family health, they are most directly implicated in policies which promote personal and parental responsibility. Section 4.4 returns to a theme developed in the Introduction to the book and examines the role of women in health policies which emphasise the responsibilities of individuals, families and communities.

Sexual divisions not only influence the organisation of women's work on behalf of their families. Sexual divisions are linked to family health in a second and more direct way. Chapter 5 explores their influence upon the health of the carers and upon the health of children in female-headed households.

4.2 GENDER DIVISIONS AND WOMEN'S RESPONSIBILITIES IN THE HOME

The greater participation of married women in paid employment has been a major feature of the post-war economy. However, while women increasingly share with men the burden of making money, housework and childcare are still largely women's work. A series of studies have found that changes in the employment activity of married women have not been matched by any substantial sharing of domestic activities between men and women (Land, 1981). Whether in paid employment or not, women retain the major responsibilities for family health. However, when the mother is unable to care for the family and in need of care herself, there is evidence to suggest that fathers, alone or with the support of kin, shoulder the burden. When mothers are in part-time employment, the father takes care of their pre-school children (Burnell and Wadsworth, 1981:72). During pregnancy and childbirth, fathers are the most significant sources of care for mothers and their children (Bell, McKee and Priestley, 1983:40). These studies also highlight the importance of kin in supporting the family when the mother cannot provide full-time care. Women's kinship networks (the mother's mother, mother-in-law and sister) are particularly important, and are generally rated as more useful than friendship networks (Argyle, 1983). While we tend to think of the elderly as consumers of family services, they also play a vital role as the producers of services (Land, 1981:21). Like other members of the family, grandparents provide baby-sitting, day care and help during illness: they also provide money and accommodation for parents with young children.

Since the mid-1970s, the increasing participation of women in paid employment has been overtaken by another change in the British economy. The official rate of unemployment in Britain climbed from 2% in June 1973 to over 12% in June 1983 (Department of Employment July Press Release). Job loss has generally been higher in manufacturing industries, which employ a high proportion of men, than in service industries, which employ a high proportion of women. As a result, men have suffered greater job losses than women. We noted above that the employment status of women does not appear to alter the division of domestic responsibilities: does the employment status of men have a more marked effect? Has the rise in male unemployment been associated with any share of domestic duties? Research is still in progress (Bell and McKee). Evidence from small-scale studies suggests that unemployed men do more around the house than their employed brothers (Collins, 1982; Nandy, 1982). But, with a few exceptions, they do not do as much as their partners. More importantly, while unemployed men take on more chores, they do not necessarily share responsibility. They help out and lend a hand, but the job remains the woman's. Further, because they are unemployed, the wife's job can become more difficult. In many families, the management of the household income and the maintenance of the family's health on social security benefits places additional demands on the carer (McKee, 1983).

He likes to be the breadwinner and that's hard on a man but the hardest bit on a woman is like managing on unemployment ... that's the biggest problem. 'Cause to me, being unemployed, I know it sounds daft, but you've got to work at being unemployed if you want to survive.
[A mother with four children, and a husband who is unemployed.][1]

Whatever the employment position of the family, it thus appears that it is typically the mother who looks after the house and looks after the children. In so doing, she is the person who takes charge of health education and training in the home. She, too, is in charge of the sick: providing care, involving professionals and implementing their advice.

The significant role played by the wife-mother as a primary agent of health behaviour in the family is becoming increasingly clear ... Whatever the measure used — illnesses incurred, medical and health services used, anticipated difficulty in using the sick role, potential impact of illness on the family or primary source of familial assistance in times of illness — the wife/mother remained the central agent of cure and care within the family complex.[2]

In general, studies indicate that women play a pivotal role in determining the health behaviour of their children, in decision-making as to use of health services, in escorting children to physicians, dentists and other sources of health services and in providing home nursing for ill children.[3]

In meeting these responsibilities, women rely on a wide range of material resources. For many families, the vital resources are likely to be in short supply. In 1981, nearly a quarter of Britain's children and their parents lived in poverty, without an income sufficient to purchase the accommodation and amenities necessary for good health (DHSS, 1983: a). However, while the economic position of many families is deteriorating, national surveys suggest that most British households have access to the resources they need for health (OPCS, 1982: a).

While the majority of families have sufficient resources, we cannot automatically assume that women have access to them. Instead, research confirms experience in recording that resources are not always allocated in line with responsibilities. Custom accords certain privileges to the male breadwinner: in terms of money, food, leisure and transport (Pahl, 1980; Pickup, 1981; Murcott, 1983). For example, national surveys record the fact that the majority (65%) of families in Britain have a car (OPCS, 1982: a). But only a minority of housewives have the use of what is — perhaps optimistically — known as the family car. Amongst most car-owning families, it is 'Daddy's car'. Less than one third (29%) of housewives have access to a car on a daily basis (Hillman, Henderson and Whalley, 1974). Like transport, other resources are not always pooled and shared equitably (see Part III).

Although these inequalities in the division of resources reflect the priority attached to male needs, inequality is not necessarily male-imposed. Surveys conducted over the last hundred years have recorded the fact that the allocation of resources is frequently instituted by the mother (Oren, 1974). As the carer, she acts as a buffer, protecting the welfare of her family by absorbing shortages herself. By cutting back on her own consumption, she is able to release additional resources for her husband and children. By reducing her needs for food and leisure, for example, a mother can provide a better diet and more attention for her children. The creation of extra resources through self-sacrifice figures strongly in the lives of families dependent on welfare benefits (Burghes, 1980; McKee, 1983). It figures strongly, too, in the lives of single parents, where it serves as a crucial strategy for 'making ends meet' (Marsden, 1973; Evason, 1980: a).

In a working class home if there is saving to be done, it is not the husband and children, but the mother who makes her meal off the scraps which remain over or 'plays with meatless bones'. One woman writes: 'I can assure you I have told my husband many times that I had had my dinner before he came in, so as there should be plenty to go round for the children and himself'.[4]

The internal distribution of resources plays an obvious but

important part in determining the quality of care that women can provide. Where the distribution is controlled by the husband/father, the women's health care role can be severely restricted. For example, in households where the family purse and the family car are in the hands of the father, the mother is unlikely to make full use of the social facilities which promote child health. Shopping areas supplying fresh food and play areas offering opportunities for exploration and adventure are likely to remain out of reach. Out of reach, too, are the medical services provided for children: child health clinics, dentists and doctors.

The question of 'who gets what' in the home has implications for the health of children. It has implications, too, for the health of mothers. In making sacrifices for the family, the health of the carer tends to suffer. These health-effects of caring are discussed in the next chapter.

4.3 GENDER DIVISIONS AND WOMEN'S PAID WORK

We have seen how a sexual division of labour operates within the home, distributing responsibilities and resources unevenly between men and women. A parallel division of labour operates within the world of paid employment. Here, too, we find 'men's work' and 'women's work', with women employed in jobs which are the market equivalent of their unpaid domestic work. Women are employed in jobs which involve traditionally female responsibilities: cleaning, cooking, clothing, caring. They are employed in jobs with few resources: job security and pay in particular are often in short supply. This section examines the position of women in the labour market and its consequences for family income.

Most women and men in Britain have paid jobs. The 1980 General Household Survey found, among those of working age, over 60% of women and 90% of men in employment. However, although most women and men are at work, the 'employment profiles' of the sexes are very different. Three differences are identified: in the jobs women and men do, in the pay they receive, and in their participation in full and part-time work.

Firstly, while men are found across the spectrum of occupations, women are concentrated in only a few industries and occupations. Over half of all female manual workers are employed in catering, cleaning, hairdressing or other personal services. Among female non-manual workers, the picture is similar, with the same proportion working in clerical and related occupations (Figure 4.1). Women's paid work matches their unpaid work: doing on a large scale for society what they traditionally have done on a small scale for their family (Huws, 1982:15).

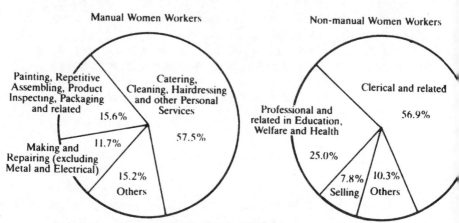

Figure 4.1: Where Women Work, 1980

Source: Department of Employment (1981) *New Earnings Survey 1980*, Table 135.

Women are not only concentrated in 'women's jobs'. They are secondly, as a result, concentrated in low-paying jobs. Analysis of the figures from the 1982 New Earnings Survey shows that women's average gross weekly pay is still less than two-thirds that of men (EOC, 1983). The marked improvement in women's pay, evident in the mid-seventies, was shortlived: women's full-time earnings are now falling relative to men (Low Pay Review, 1983:23).

Women's earnings have suffered in the recession along with those of the low-paid in general. 'Low pay' is defined and measured in a variety of ways: in terms of the level of supplementary benefit and family income supplement, for example, or in relation to average earnings. The trade unions usually consider anyone earning less than two-thirds the average adult male manual wage to be low-paid. Although derived in different ways, these measures converge around a weekly income in 1983 of £90 gross (or £2.30 an hour). This is the figure taken by the Low Pay Unit as their definition of low pay.

According to government figures, from the 1982 New Earnings Survey, the lowest paid jobs are in hairdressing, catering and cleaning and in clothing and educational services. These are industries where women predominate. Reflecting this, we find that 52% of full-time women workers are low-paid, compared with 15% of full-time male workers (Table 4.1). Put in more concrete terms, this means that a mother contributing to the family wage by working full-time as a hairdresser would earn gross, without overtime, £56.00 a week (1982 figures).

Table 4.1: Estimated Numbers and Proportion of Adult Workers Earning Low Wages, April 1982

	Including overtime		*Excluding overtime*	
	million	*%*	*million*	*%*
Full-time males	1·0	10·1	1·4	15·1
Full-time females	2·2	50·0	2·3	51·9
Part-time males	0·2	33·7	—	—
Part-time females	2·3	64·6	—	—

Source: Department of Employment *New Earnings Survey 1982* reproduced in Byrne, D., Pond, C. & Sullivan, J. (1983) *Low Wages in Britain*, p.5.

There is a third important feature of women's employment. Women are disproportionately represented among part-time workers. Part-time work has been increasing in significance over the last two decades, and one in five of the employed labour force now works part-time. Part-time work, however, is predominantly women's work: 90% of part-time workers are women. Thus while only 4% of men work part-time, 40% of women do (Rimmer and Popay, 1982: 2).

The main reason why women choose or find themselves restricted to part-time jobs is because of their home responsibilities. These responsibilities often add up to a life-cycle of caring — caring first for children, then for elderly relatives and finally for elderly spouses. However, it is their responsibility for caring for children which has the first and lasting impact upon their employment profiles. Most women give up work before their first baby is born. When they return to work, they do so on a part-time basis. This pattern of employment is reflected in Tables 4.2 and

4.3. Table 4.2 records the economic activity of women in and out of marriage, while Table 4.3 reveals the extent to which it is motherhood, rather than marriage, which marks the turning-point in women's employment. As Table 4.3 indicates, 70% of mothers with pre-school children are not employed. Among mothers with school-aged children, only a third are without part-time or full-time work.

Table 4.2: Economic Activity of Women aged 16-59 by Marital Status: Great Britain, 1980 (number in sample = 8821)

Marital status	Working full-time %	Working part-time %	Not working %
Single (unmarried)	61	4	34
Separated, divorced and widowed	38	24	38
Married	26	33	40
All Women	34	26	39

Source: OPCS (1982) *General Household Survey 1980*, Table 5.2, p.94.

Table 4.3: Economic Activity of Mothers aged 16-59 with Dependent Children: Great Britain, 1980 (number in sample = 4175)

Age of youngest dependent child	Working full-time %	Working part-time %	Not Working %
Under 5	7	23	70
5 and over	23	44	33
All ages	17	36	46

Source: OPCS (1982) *General Household Survey 1980*, Table 5.4, p.95.

Table 4.4: Employment Status of Lone Mothers with Dependent Children
Combined General Household Survey figures for 1979-81

Age of youngest child	Working full-time %	Working part-time %	Not working %
Under 5	12	12	76
5 and over	27	31	41
All ages	23	25	51

Source: Popay, J., Rimmer, L. & Rossiter (1983) *One Parent Families*, Study Commission on the Family, p.49. Crown Copyright.

Given the fact that it is mothers and not fathers who take primary responsibility for childcare, we would not expect the arrival of children to have the same impact on male employment. The data bear out this expectation. In two parent families, men with children are no more likely to be unemployed than men without children. In fact, the evidence suggests that married fathers are under-represented among the unemployed (Rimmer & Popay, 1982). However, the incidence of unemployment is greater for heads of large families and for men who are divorced or separated (Layard, Piachaud and Stewart 1978:90; Daniel, 1981:11.30). With the current rise in youth unemployment, age rather than family commitments may emerge as the more important factor protecting men in employment. In a recent study of fathers, unemployment was heavily concentrated among those under twenty-five, with the younger mothers tending to be married to men who were unemployed (Bell, McKee, Priestley, 1983:20).

The arrival of children is associated with longer working hours for married men in employment. As women give up their paid jobs to care for the children, the burden of income-production shifts on to the man. Reduced to one wage earner at a time of greater financial commitments, young fathers take on more work outside the home. Evidence suggests that they are particularly likely to do more overtime (Moss, 1980).

While children do not appear to have a marked effect on the careers of married men, we might expect a more profound change in the employment patterns of lone fathers. George and Wilding, in their study of nearly 600 lone fathers, found that childcare responsibilities reduced the earning power of their respondents. Take-home pay fell in the years which followed their wife's death or departure, particularly among manual workers (George and Wilding, 1972:87). For these fathers, the loss of income was directly linked to their changed domestic circumstances, with family responsibilities forcing them to take lower-paid jobs and to restrict their overtime. In addition, about a third of the sample (35%) had had to give up work at some stage to look after their children full-time. A similar pattern, of interrupted employment and reduced income for a significant minority of lone fathers, has been uncovered in more recent studies (Hipgrave, 1982).

However, while many lone fathers have problems reconciling wage-earning with childcare, their employment patterns are not so severely affected by parenthood as are those of women with children (See Tables 4.3 and 4.4). Instead, despite the problems, lone fathers tend to have employment profiles similar to those of their married brothers. In aggregate terms, neither the working hours nor the earnings of the two groups appear to differ substantially (Popay, Rimmer and Rossiter, 1983: 532).

The distinctive pattern of women's employment — their concentration in part-time jobs in a restricted range of low-paying occupations — is associated with what we earlier identified as a dual labour market. This segmented labour market is characterised by a primary sector of what are commonly regarded as 'good jobs'. These jobs are typically secure, well-paid and satisfying. In the secondary sector, by contrast, employment tends to be insecure, poorly-paid and repetitive. It offers a wage-packet but not a career. The available evidence suggests that many women, and women with children in particular, are restricted to the secondary labour market because of their family responsibilities. The low-grade and low-paid work they secure there often mirrors and compounds the pressures they experience at home (Shimmin, McNally and Liff, 1981; Pollert, 1981:118-20).

The existence of a dual labour market limits the contribution that women (and a significant number of men) can make to family income. In two parent families, women's earnings are often critical in keeping the family above the poverty line. It is calculated that, without the earnings of women, the number of families in poverty would increase fourfold (CPRS, 1980). However, it is in one parent families that the economic consequences of the dual labour market are most apparent.

Single parent families, are, by definition, one wage-earner families. Further, in most families, this one wage earner is a woman. Their potential for increasing family income through paid employment is thus restricted both by the number and sex of the adults in the household. In addition, there is evidence to suggest that lone mothers are further disadvantaged in the labour market. A DHSS study of lone mothers on Family Income Supplement suggested that they were lower paid than the total population of working women. Their overall average earnings were about 70% of those of full-time female workers (Nixon, 1979:71).

There is conclusive evidence that women tend to be worse off than men on virtually all indices of economic status. Households headed by women are, for example, 4½ times as likely as those headed by men to be in poverty ... The poverty of lone mothers is particularly striking.[5]

Such evidence suggests that while employment rescues many lone mothers from extreme need, the wages they are able to earn rarely secure more than a modest standard of living for their families. The low wages available to women were identified by the Finer Report as a major factor in perpetuating the poverty of one parent families. The Finer Committee argued strongly for policies which improved the employment opportunities for women, and for the day-care facilities to enable lone mothers to take advantage of them. A series of studies have noted the lack of day-care for the children of working mothers (Hunt, Fox and Morgan 1973; Jackson and Jackson, 1979). With the most common arrangement found in two parent families — care by the father — not available, the problem for lone mothers is particularly serious. The bulk of substitute care is provided for lone mothers on an informal basis by friends, relatives and neighbours (Evason, 1980:a; Letts, 1983). Most of this informal care is also unpaid. Child minders and statutory workplace provision meet only a small proportion of lone mothers' need for day care.

Day care is important not only in enabling lone mothers to work and improve the economic circumstances in which they and their children live. Day care has a more direct relation to family health. Day care services for children can protect both parents and children from the extremes of social isolation found among a minority of single parents (Evason, 1980:a:46). The question of the health of the carer is raised again in Chapter 5.

This section has focussed on the complex relationship between sex and employment status. It has highlighted the disadvantaged position of women in the labour market and its role in family poverty. Women's position in the labour market is seen as directly linked to the poverty of one parent families, as Finer noted. The low pay of women also keeps many two parent families in the margins of poverty (McNay and Pond, 1980). However, without their earnings, the health and standard of living of families would deteriorate sharply.

Domestic work in the family and paid work for the family does not exhaust women's responsibilities for family health. Women's health care role is receiving increasing attention in a third arena: that of the welfare state.

4.4　GENDER DIVISIONS AND SOCIAL POLICY

The division of labour between men and women provides the backcloth against which health work in the home is organised. It provides, too, the context in which women seek paid employment to improve the living standards of their family. In this final section, we consider a third important spin-off of sexual divisions for family health: their impact upon government policy in the field of health and welfare.

The pervasive influence of gender in the design and delivery of services is not immediately apparent. Policy documents released over the last decade have emphasised that everyone has a part to play in combating ill-health. The vocabulary is explicitly and unequivocally gender-neutral. It is not women but individuals, familes and communities who are encouraged to take more responsibility for their health. Health is everybody's business.

We all have a personal responsibility for our own health. We also have a duty to help one another . . . The prevention of mental and physical ill-health is a prime objective, and an area in which the individual has clear responsibilities . . .

It has been a major policy objective for many years to foster and develop community care for the main client groups — elderly, mentally ill, mentally handicapped and disabled people and children.[6]

The primary sources of support and care for elderly people are informal and voluntary . . . They are irreplaceable. It is the role of public authorities to sustain, and where necessary, develop — but never to displace — such support and care. Care *in* the community must increasingly mean care *by* the community.[7]

Given that women, at present, carry the burden of concern and care for the health of the family, an emphasis on health as the collective responsibility of all people would indeed mark a radical departure in government policy. However, the evidence suggests that the policies of preventative health and community care do not so much challenge the existing health roles of women, as presume them. Policies which emphasise informal support and voluntary care have been found to translate into a practice of support and care by women. Abrams notes in his survey of community care that 'the bulk of helping that is reported as community care turns out at closer scrutiny to be kin care' (1977:134). Reflecting this fact, the Equal Opportunities Commission in its survey of elderly and handicapped dependents found that 'most carers are women ... and most women will at some time in their lives become carers' (1982:4).

A parallel process is apparent in the field of preventive health. Here, a major theme concerns what parents can and should do for child health. In supporting parents, health education aims to give them an accurate and realistic picture of what child-rearing entails. In addition, it has the objective of making parents more informed and responsible about their children's development by pointing out hazards to child health which they can control themselves. In realising these objectives, programmes of attitude and behaviour change have been instituted. However, again, in the translation from principle into practice, men tend to fade from view. The focus shifts from *parents*, to detail what *mothers* can do to promote child health. Thus, while parents are encouraged to involve themselves in the experience and re-sponsibilities of family life (DHSS, 1973; DHSS, 1977), fathers find the opportunities for involvement are restricted by their employment commitments (Bell, McKee, Priestley, 1983). Sim-ilarly, while preparation for parenthood is seen as an exercise for both parents-to-be, its organisation tends to reinforce the idea that parenthood is for women only (Graham, 1979:a). It is generally mothers who are urged to attend early and regularly for antenatal care, to bring their babies to the child health clinic for immunisation and check-ups, to ensure their home is safe and their supervision sufficient to prevent accidental injury. Fathers who wish to be parents too can find themselves marginalised by the way in which health services are delivered to their children (Strong, 1979; Brown, 1982).

When a couple did attend a (paediatric) clinic together, staff placed fathers in a subordinate position to their spouses. Questions were asked directly of the mothers and, though fathers sometimes added their own comments to which staff might reply, they normally returned to the mother for their next question ... Fathers who had a lot to say had usually to interrupt a running conversation. The structure of the situation automatically defined them as rude and in-considerate: a fact which such fathers usually acknowledged with grins and apologies.[8]

It is not only in preventive programmes of child health that responsibility devolves on to mothers. Men and women can find themselves with different roles, and different responsibilities, in programmes designed to improve adult health. For example, while coronary heart disease is seen as a problem which primarily affects men, the obligation to 'look after yourself' can bypass them and fall to their wives. Identified as the carers within the family, they are also seen as the primary agents of change in health attitudes and behaviour.

It is highly unlikely that you will persuade your husband to give up smoking if you smoke yourself. Show your husband that you intend to deal firmly with the smoking habit. The sensible wife will first decide whether her husband should lose weight and then plan his menu accordingly. Without cutting them out altogether, cut down on starchy foods like bread, potatoes, sugar, breakfast cereal, spaghetti, jam, cakes, puddings and sweets ... Encourage him to take the dog for a walk in the evenings, and to take regular exercise at the weekends. The more time you can find to join him on walks or gardening, the less he will feel that exercise is something to which he is being 'subjected'. Sports and games are also useful. You could, for example, play tennis regularly at weekends with your children or with a neighbouring couple, or else take up golf ...

Let your husband talk about his worries, and wherever possible take the work from him — draft letters, pay bills, arrange for the plumber to come yourself ...[9]

The changes recommended to improve the health of husbands and children are usually presented as a list of 'simple precautions'. When listed separately, such precautions as not smoking in pregnancy or taking up sport may indeed appear simple and straightforward. However, the cumulative impact of such 'dos' and 'don'ts' can be more disruptive. Together, the recommended changes can constitute a radical restructuring of daily life. For example, pregnant women are currently advised to improve their diet, watch their weight, cut down on alcohol, stop smoking, give up paid employment and seek regular medical check-ups for the sake of their baby. Similarly, in the passage above, the recommendations for reducing the risk of heart attack demand a new diet for the family and a new timetable for the carer to incorporate the items designed to keep the man of the house fit and healthy. Such advice presumes that it is a woman's wish (and duty) to shape her own life-style around the needs of her husband. It presumes, too, that she had the ability to achieve such changes. It assumes that women can act autonomously within the family, insulated from economic and social constraints. Yet, research suggests that many women do not have the degree of control over their life-style in which such advice is meaningful and practical (Cullen and Phelps, 1975:62-3; Pill and Stott, 1982).

This question of choice and control is central to current policies in the field of family life. It is one to which later chapters return. Here, we have only indicated the particular and often invisible way in which women are implicated in these policies. Community care, self-help and parental responsibility, within both two and one parent families, are not experiences uniformly distributed between the sexes. Instead, the burden of these caring obligations is shouldered by women. Carrying these heavy health responsibilities limits women's opportunities in the labour market. As we noted earlier in the chapter, low-paid workers are predominantly women workers: part-time work, too, is a euphemism for women's work. Taking responsibility for family health thus reduces women's capacity to earn the material resources necessary for family health. It also appears to reduce their command over the resources secured through their husband's job: the family car, for example, typically remains in the husband's hands. The fact that women's health responsibilities severely limit their access to health resources may appear paradoxical, but it provides the basis on which care is organised in the home. Recognition of this fact is thus central to an understanding of how families work for health. It is also central to an understanding of the health of the health workers: the main subject of Chapter 5.

NOTES

1. McKee, L. (1983) 'Wives and the Recession', University of Aston, p.11.
2. Litman, T.J. (1974) 'The Family as a Basic Unit in Health and Medical Care', *Social Science and Medicine*, Vol.8, p.505.
3. Carpenter, E.S. (1980) 'Children's Health Care and the Changing Role of Women', *Medical Care*, Vol.18, 12, p.1210.
4. Women's Co-operative Guild (1915) *Maternity: Letters from Working Women*, p.5.
5. Brown, M. & Madge, N. (1982) *Despite the Welfare State*, p.58.
6. DHSS (1981: a) *Care in Action*, pp.1, 11 and 12.
7. DHSS (1981: b) *Growing Older*, Cmnd. 8173, para. 1.9.
8. Strong, P. (1979) *The Ceremonial Order of the Clinic: Patients, Doctors and Medical Bureaucracies*, pp.61-2.
9. Flora Project for Heart Disease Prevention, (undated) *Coronary Disease: How to Protect Your Family*.

5 Gender Divisions:
The Impact on Health

5.1 INTRODUCTION

This chapter, like the previous one, is concerned with the division between men's work and women's work and its influence on family health. Chapter 4 examined the impact of sexual divisions on women's work, both in and beyond the family: here the focus is more directly on the question of health and illness. The chapter looks at two areas in which the traditional roles of men and women are known to affect individual health. It considers, firstly, the differences between men and women in mortality and morbidity. Singled out for discussion is the apparent vulnerability of mothers with young children to mental illness. It looks, secondly, at the differences in the health of women and children in one and two parent families.

The main sections of the chapter thus address the following areas: sex differences in health; mental illness among women; the health of the carers, and, in the final section, health in one and two parent families.

5.2 PERSPECTIVES ON SEX DIFFERENCES IN HEALTH

The marked sex differences in health experiences were summarised in Chapter 3 (see Figure 3.3 and 3.7 and 3.8). Women live longer than men and have a lower rate of mortality in all age groups (Brown and Madge, 1982: 111). Despite their greater longevity, women are more likely to suffer from both chronic and acute disorders. They also make more use of medical services, particularly those of their GP.

Patterns of mortality and morbidity are increasingly being related to life-styles and living conditions. Differences in the health experiences of men and women, like differences between the social classes, are seen to reflect differences in the way that people live. In particular, sex differences are seen to reflect differences in the working conditions of men and women. In general terms, it appears that it is the particular kind and pace of men's work which makes men, as a sex, more vulnerable to premature death. Similarly, it is the kind and pace of work which women do which makes women more vulnerable to ill-health.

The relation between life-style, or more accurately work-style, and health is clearly complex. The class patterns of health, outlined in Chapter 3, suggest that the class structure has a consistent and negative influence on the health of working-class families, resulting in their higher rates of morbidity and mortality. Sexual divisions do not operate in such a uni-directional way, serving to protect the health of one sex and undermine the health of the other. Instead, the sex patterns of health suggest that cross-cutting forces are in operation, which protect and undermine the health of both sexes in different ways.

The task of understanding these complex forces is still a long way from completion. Certain tendencies within this area of research, however, can be noted. Research into sex differences tends to be sex-specific. Moreover, because the orientation of men-based and women-based investigations tends to be different, their findings cannot always be compared.

The gap in life expectancy between men and women is one of the most distinctive features of human health in the advanced societies. The risk of death for men in each occupational class is almost twice that of women, the cumulative product of health inequalities between the sexes during the whole lifetime. It suggests that gender and class exert highly significant but different influences on the quality and duration of life in modern society.[1]

Most of the research on the health of men has centred on the occupational sphere. It is their attitudes to, and relationship with, the labour market which is seen as the major determinant of their health. Thus, a man's personality and employment status have been identified as the crucial variables. However, it is difficult to establish whether these factors operate as causes or effects of poor health. Where men demonstrate certain psychological tendencies and 'coronary prone' behaviours, stress-related disorders tend to be higher than among more sanguine male workers, but the causal processes are hard to disentangle (Review Body, 1981). Among unemployed men, too, health appears to deteriorate, although again the data are equivocal. An analysis of data from the OPCS longitudinal study, initiated in 1971, suggests that mortality rates are markedly higher among unemployed than employed men (Hakim, 1982:446). Adverse health-effects of unemployment have been noted, too, in other studies (College, 1981). However, data from the DHSS cohort study of the unemployed found no evidence that health deteriorated during the time when men were out of work (Ramsden and Smee 1981:399). The majority of those becoming unemployed appeared to be relatively healthy and remained so throughout the first year following registration. Shifting from physical to psychological health, attention has been drawn particularly to the role of unemployment in suicide, the rates of which have been increasing steadily since the mid-seventies (Hakim, 1982:447). Unemployment, but not psychiatric illness, is a characteristic of about half of male parasuicides, and suicide deaths are highest among young men in social class five, the group most vulnerable to unemployment (ibid). There is evidence, too, that the threat of unemployment can produce symptoms of stress among those still at work (Dooley and Catalano, 1980).

In this concern with the occupational identity of men, the wider consequences of employment for the family have been neglected. As Hakim notes, there is a tendency to personalise unemployment, regarding it as a problem for the unemployed themselves (Hakim, 1982:459). As a result the impact of men's work and men's health on the family has gone largely unexplored. Yet we know that when the man of the house is unemployed, the health of children suffers. Rates of admissions to hospital, in particular, are significantly higher among young children of the unemployed. When social class is controlled for, hospital admissions rates are double those found among the children of families in employment (Brennan and Lancashire, 1978). Other studies suggest that parental unemployment during childhood has long-term health effects, extending well into adulthood (Burr and Sweetnam, 1980). The health effects of male unemployment on women's health has received less attention. However, it is known that women often give up or postpone their search for work when their husbands lose their jobs (Hakim, 1982; McKee, 1983). In such circumstances, women must cope both with the psychological consequences of their own and their partner's unemployment and with the practical task of managing the family budget on a sharply reduced income.

While research on men's health has concerned itself with the occupational domain, research on women's health traditionally has paid primary attention to the domestic domain. It is women's position in the home which is seen to hold the key to women's health. In highlighting the health-effects of women's domestic role, it is the social rather than material aspects of domesticity which have been stressed. The quality of women's health is seen as crucially linked to the quality of their relationships with their partner and children. Their physical and mental health, in turn, is regarded to be a significant influence on their children. Thus, studies of children identify the mental state of the mother as a key variable in their analyses of behaviour problems and developmental delay. Significantly, the mental state of the father is often not recorded or used in the search for statistically significant relationships (see, for example, Richman, Stevenson and Graham, 1982; Wilson and Herbert, 1978).

Recently the narrow focus upon women's relationships within the home has begun to broaden. A number of studies have examined the influence of paid as well as unpaid labour on women's health (Stellman, 1977; Shimmin, McNally and Liff, 1981). In so doing, they have addressed the effects which the physical conditions of women's lives — within and beyond the home — have upon their health. Housing conditions, for example, have long been known to have a more marked effect on women and pre-school children than on other members of the family, since they spend more of their time at home (Spring Rice, 1939: 13-14). Dampness, overcrowding and lack of basic amenities all create health problems, particularly for women and young children (Doyal, 1983: 28). Men, too, have a physical presence which can cause ill-health in women. Husbands and fathers can carry dangerous substances from work into the home, as the evidence of asbestosis among the wives and children of asbestos workers starkly demonstrates (BSSRS, 1979: 29). Marital violence, also, is known to be a cause of physical injury and emotional distress among women (Dobash and Dobash, 1982: 197). These violent attacks are typically witnessed by the children (ibid.: 198). With assaults by men on their wives representing 25% of all violent crime (CIS, 1981: 4), violence in marriage is clearly a significant, but unrecorded, source of ill-health among mothers, and their children.

Although men also suffer on occasions from the effects of violence, domestic violence against women does have its own particular characteristics. Most importantly, it tends to be sustained over a considerable period of time, since the structure of marriage makes it difficult for women to either get help or to leave. Furthermore, the violence often involves children, making it an even more devastating experience for the woman and the result is likely to be both physical and psychological damage — usually of a deep and long-lasting kind.[2]

Environmental hazards are found not only in the home. As for men, the working conditions of women in employment can place their health at risk. Moreover, since women in the labour force are concentrated in particular industries, they are exposed to specific health risks which men may avoid. Secretarial work, hotel and catering work and nursing, for example, have their own distinctive patterns of occupational disease (Stellman, 1977: 81-138).

Broadening our perspective to include the social and material conditions of women's work inside and outside the home can enhance our understanding of physical health. It has much to contribute, also, to our understanding of mental health. It is in the rates of mental illness that the sex differences are most pronounced. It is here, therefore, that research has concentrated.

5.3 WOMEN AND MENTAL ILLNESS

More women than men are classified as having neurotic and depressive disorders, they are more likely to be prescribed psychotropic drugs and to be admitted to a psychiatric hospital. Admission rates to psychiatric hospitals are over one third higher for women and rates of admission for depressive and neurotic disorders show an even more pronounced sex difference (Table 5.1). One in ten men, but as many as one in five women, will take tranquillisers or sleeping pills during the course of a year. The greater susceptibility of women to depression is common to all industrialised countries (Weissman and Klerman, 1977). However, there is considerable controversy about the meaning of these sex differences.

It has been suggested that the higher rates of depression and neurosis among women result from the roles and responsibilities that women perform: their lives are inherently more depressing and stress-producing. There is considerable support for this view, with the rates of depression closely linked to the distribution of

Table 5.1: Mental Illness Hospitals and Units (1979):
Admissions by Sex and Diagnostic Group: Selected Diagnoses Only

	Male	Female
'Male disorders'		
Alcoholism and alcoholic psychosis	8,919	3,840
Drug dependence	726	376
'Female disorders'		
Depressive psychoses	6,514	14,681
Psychoneuroses	5,582	12,552
Senile dementia	4,292	8,528
Other psychoses	4,394	7,453
Other psychiatric conditions	15,333	29,083
All diagnoses	68,108	101,202

Source: DHSS (1982) *Health and Personal Social Services Statistics,*
  Table 9.4, p. 114.

disadvantage. Brown and Harris, in their study of *The Social Origins of Depression*, found the highest rates of undiagnosed depression among working-class women who were full-time (and often housebound) carers. Among working-class women with a child under six, one third (31%) were found to have what would be clinically regarded as a psychiatric disorder (Brown and Harris, 1978: 151).

Particular aspects of women's lives have been identified in the causal chain linking social environment to psychiatric disorder. Poverty, poor housing, unemployment and isolation have been repeatedly found to be strongly associated with depression. A study of 800 families in Waltham Forest underlines the importance of these environmental influences (Richman, Stevenson and Graham, 1982). The study highlights the importance of housing conditions and financial stress in fuelling depression. Mothers with pre-school children living in council-rented accommodation were more at risk than owner-occupiers; living on the fourth floor and above was also significantly related to the presence of depression (ibid.: 166-7). Mothers living in tower-blocks have also been found to report higher rates of depression in other studies (Littlewood and Tinker, 1981). Financial stress, as measured by debt and difficulty in meeting bills, has also been linked to depression among mothers of young children (Richman, Stevenson, & Graham, 1982: 168), as has unemployment among both women and their partners (Brown and Harris, 1978:237; Rimmer and Popay, 1982:79-80). Significantly, male workers who are unemployed are also more vulnerable to psychiatric disorder than those in employment (College, 1981; Kelvin, 1981; Hakim, 1982). While unemployment increases vulnerability, employment does not always act to protect an individual against depression. Crucial is the nature of the work itself. As the authors of the Waltham Forest study note 'at worst, work can mean long or anti-social hours in a low-paid job in addition to a heavy load of housework ... at best, however, a woman's job can provide her with high status, good working conditions, an alternative source of satisfaction and social relationships, flexible hours to match her family needs, as well as sufficient pay to get help in the home. These advantages and disadvantages for individuals may well cancel out when a total population is studied' (Richman, Stevenson and Graham, 1982: 169). Reflecting this cancelling effect perhaps, their study found a definite but not significant relationship between unemployment and maternal depression.

Material deprivation and unemployment are not the only factors identified in the aetiology of depression. Research has also underlined the importance of social isolation. Brown and Harris (1978) suggested that a confiding relationship with one's spouse offered protection against depression: other researchers have stressed the role of supportive relationships in general (Gavron, 1966; Graham and McKee, 1980:24; Evason, 1980:a). In our survey of 200 mothers with young children, over 40% reported themselves to be lonely five months after the birth of their baby and over a half had not got out without their children (Graham and McKee, 1980: 24). In a study of 700 lone parents, most of whom had school-aged children, a similar picture emerges. Evason found that one third of the lone parents felt themselves to be very isolated, and nearly one half had not had an evening out without the children in the last month (Evason, 1980: a: 51). Both studies found a significant association between social isolation and depression.

Women's greater susceptibility to nervous disorders may result not simply from the stress-inducing conditions in which many women live. It may reflect the particular way in which others respond to stress in women (Smith and David, 1974). The greater susceptibility of women to depression and neurosis may reflect the diagnostic habits of doctors, social workers and psychiatrists.

Thus, for example, what passes as overwork or 'job burn-out' in men, may be identified as depression in women. Diagnosis is typically followed by a prescription: in a study of drug use in Oxfordshire, psychotropics accounted for almost one-fifth of all prescriptions. 10% of men and 21% of women receiving prescribed drugs had at least one psychotropic prescription during the year (Skegg, Doll and Perry, 1977). Repeat prescriptions are an important feature of psychotropic drug use, particularly among women. The habitual use of drugs such as diazepam (valium) has promoted researchers to look at the meaning of tranquillisers for those who depend upon them. In so doing, they have shifted the focus from the sex-specific way in which professionals respond to stress in their clients, and examined the sex-specific way in which women express stress (Baker Miller, 1976). Alcoholism and crime, for example, are more typically male responses: rates of admission to psychiatric hospital because of alcoholism and rates of criminal convictions are significantly higher among men than women. In fact, if crime and psychiatric disorders (including alcoholism) are treated together, the sex differences in mental illness largely disappear (Brown and Madge, 1982:112).

If women tend to vent their feelings of stress in more silent and self-effacing ways than men, then their high rate of psychotropic drug use takes on a new significance. Research suggests that tranquillisers do not so much cure depression as enable their users to cope with the responsibilities which trigger it. The effects of the diazepams appear particularly suited to the role-strains of domestic life, enabling women 'to maintain themselves in roles that they found difficult or intolerable without them' (Cooperstock and Lennard, 1979:335).

I take it [valium] to protect the family from my irritability because the kids are kids. I don't think it's fair for me to start yelling at them because their normal activity is bothering me ... So I take the valium to keep me calm ... peace and calm. That's what my husband wants because frankly the kids get on his nerves, too ... when I blow my top I am told to settle down. When he does it, it's perfectly alright.[3]

While differing in emphasis, these perspectives on mental illness acknowledge that sex differences in health, like class differences in health, are largely environmental in origin. It is accepted that it is the social and physical environment that men inhabit which exposes them to dangerous accidents and episodes of violence. Similarly, it is the social and physical world of women which makes them vulnerable to chronic ill-health and mental stress. The social causes are clearly complex, and combine in a contradictory way to increase the vulnerability of women to illness (mental and physical) and men to death. However, as the research reported in this section indicates, we are beginning to understand at least some of the factors involved. What emerges from the evidence is a paradox. The evidence suggests that ill-health in women stems, directly or indirectly, from the health-work they do for others. Promoting health in the family, it seems, involves its own occupational hazards.

5.4   PERSPECTIVES ON THE HEALTH OF THE CARERS

Because of women's role as the family caretakers, research on women's health provides valuable information on the health experience of those who care for the family. Thus, in describing women's health experiences, researchers have documented, intentionally or inadvertently, the health experiences of carers. In the research referenced in the previous section, the health effects of caring are typically of secondary interest: the main focus of the studies is upon the health of women-qua-women. In other studies, the concern is more explicitly with the health of the health-worker: their findings derive from and apply to both women and men who find themselves as the primary carers in the home.

Taken together, these studies on women and the carers highlight the poor health of Britain's informal health workers. For example, the 1930s study of *Working Class Wives* (Spring Rice, 1939) found an iceberg of unreported chronic illness among the 1,250 women who participated in her survey. Similarly, contemporary studies of those who care for the young, the old and the handicapped report high rates of ill-health (Bayley, 1973; EOC, 1982).

A vast gulf stretches between the standard of physical fitness demanded by the medical profession and the mere absence of sickness and disabling disease which is the criterion of health accepted by the working mother. She firmly believes that her home and family would collapse if her work was interrupted by a sojourn at the hospital, or even by the necessity of lying down or resting in bed for a few hours a day and she therefore refuses to admit that she is ill.[4]

Mental strain is a particularly common side-effect of caring. As detailed in the previous section, high rates of mental stress are found among informal health workers. Spring Rice noted that emotional exhaustion was widespread among the mothers in her sample, with tiredness and stress 'accepted with the same resignation as getting old' (Spring Rice, 1939:69). More recently, surveys of motherhood have reported the ubiquity of feelings of tiredness, loneliness and depression among those who care for young children (Richman, 1976; Graham and McKee, 1980; Hipgrave 1982). Similarly, the Equal Opportunities Commission (1982) found that while caring is physically arduous, it is the emotional demands which take the heaviest toll on the carer. The study which put figures on these feelings is *The Social Origins of Depression* (Brown and Harris, 1978). The incidence of depression among working-class women suggests that where the inequalities of class combine with those of gender, depression indeed appears to be an occupational hazard of caring.

As we noted in Chapter 3, the divisions of class and gender combine in ways which are particularly disadvantageous for one parent families. It is the health experiences of these families which are discussed in the final section of this chapter.

5.5 HEALTH IN ONE AND TWO PARENT FAMILIES

An individual's sex has a direct and measurable link with health, with men and women reporting different rates of illness and disability. Data suggest that the influence of gender works indirectly, too, shaping health through household structure. Two parent households appear to have different experiences of health than one parent households. This section reviews the evidence on health and family structure.

As we saw in Chapter 3, much research remains to be done on the relation between social class and family health. However, by comparison, the systematic study of the influence of household structure on health has hardly begun. Without such studies, we will not know whether the clear and unequivocal relationship which exists between occupational class and health exists also for family structure. National data on perinatal mortality are suggestive. Babies born to unsupported mothers, who have no man to draw them into the occupational class structure, are the most vulnerable to perinatal death. The perinatal mortality rate for illegitimate babies is nearly twice that of babies born in social class one (16.9 per 1,000 births compared with 9.7 per 1,000 births in 1980).

While data on perinatal mortality provides some indication of the impact of family structure on the health of new-born babies, there are no equivalent national data on health experiences during childhood. There are no national data either, on the health experiences of single parents. The General Household Survey does not provide an analysis of morbidity by marital status. The small numbers of respondents in one parent families and the heterogeneity of their family situations prevent any valid analysis of the impact of household structure on health (personal communication, OPCS, 1983).

Faced with this dearth of current national data, we must rely on the cohort studies of child health and development (described in Chapter 3.1). Ferri (1976) followed up the children in the 1958 National Child Development Study living in one parent families. But the most recent cohort data derive from the 1970 British Birth Survey five-year follow-up study, the CHES study. As part of this study, Burnell and Wadsworth have made a separate analysis of the data on one parent families (Burnell and Wadsworth, 1981 and 1982; Wadsworth, Burnell, Taylor and Butler, 1983). Child accidents were included in their analysis. Accidents, it was noted earlier, are the largest single cause of childhood mortality and the one in which the influence of environment is at its strongest (see Figure 3.2). The rate of (non-fatal) childhood

Table 5.2: Accidents and Hospital Admissions After Accidents: The Influence of Family Structure, Great Britain, 1975

Family type	Number	Percentage of pre-school children with one or more accident	Hospital admission after Accident
Two parent	2,482	42·7	5·8
Step family	342	52·6	10·8
One parent	716	47·3	10·3

Source: Wadsworth, J., Burnell, I., Taylor, B. and Butler, N. (1983) 'Family type and accidents in pre-school children', *Journal of Epidemiology and Community Heatlh*, 37, 2, p. 101.

accidents can thus serve as a barometer of material and social disadvantage; between the social classes and between one and two parent families.

The 1975 follow-up survey confirms that children in one parent families are more likely to have accidents than those in two parent families. They are also more likely to be admitted to hospital after an accident (Table 5.2).

While differences in the incidence of accidents are apparent between one and two parent families, they are not marked. Children in one parent families have an accident rate 10% higher than that found in two parent families; a difference which should be seen in the context of the five-fold difference in the rate of fatal accidents between children in social classes one and five (Mac-Farlane and Fox, 1978). Further, the highest rates of all were found in the 1975 follow-up study among children in step families. 53% of their parents reported an accident in the first five years of their lives.

Given the greater environmental hazards facing children in one parent families (outlined in Chapters 2 and 3), we need, perhaps, to highlight the relatively low rate of accidents among these children. An important factor here is the findings from other studies of child accidents in the home. This suggests that evenings and weekends, when both parents and other adults are present, are high-risk times for children (RCGP, 1982:4). At such times, 'vigilance is weakened when parents are distracted by the company of other adults. The adults were busy with other chores, cooking, talking or watching television' (Littlewood and Tinker, 1981:34). Children in one parent families may thus be protected by the fact that they have fewer adults looking after them. Further evidence suggests that lone parents are particularly vigilant in the supervision of their children (Weiss, 1979).

Turning from the health of children to that of their parents, the CHES follow-up survey again provides valuable data on the position of one and two parent families. Burnell and Wadsworth examined the rates of mental stress among mothers in one and two parent households. Lone mothers were found to be more likely to experience stress than women in other family situations. 39% of the lone mothers had experienced poor mental health compared with 23% of the married mothers (Burnell and Wadsworth, 1981:75). The difference in the rates may reflect, in a profoundly personal way, the impact of social and material disadvantage on women. Significantly, the rates of mental stress were similarly high among women in step families: 35% of the women in this group reported symptoms of psychiatric illness.

Evason's study of lone parents in Northern Ireland sheds further light on the probems facing lone mothers. She found that problems with sleeping, loss of appetite, lassitude and feeling overwhelmed and helpless affected between one third and one half of her sample. About one fifth experienced three or more of these symptoms of depression most of the time. She explains the pattern of depression with reference to the variables identified in the previous section: in particular, she cites low income, unemployment and social isolation. 70% of her sample lived in poverty and 65% were unemployed. In addition, one third of the single parents had no one with whom they felt they could talk about their problems. Evason again notes the importance of social networks: relatives and friends accounted for the bulk of supportive relationships. However, one quarter of the sources of support were professional and voluntary workers. As she observes, 'doctors, social workers, health visitors, samaritans and other members of self-help groups such as Gingerbread, were clearly providing vital assistance to a minority' (Evason, 1980:a: 51). Evason also identifies important differences within the lone parent group. Lone fathers, for example, were significantly less prone to depression than separated and divorced mothers. While they were just as likely to be socially isolated, lone fathers were more likely to be employed, earning incomes which lifted them and their children out of poverty.

In our final part of the questionnaire we asked our single parents about the problems uppermost in their mind ... Ms D. is widowed with three children. 'You've got the children but you're still lonely — you could be lonely in a crowd of a million people. The children are a help. I had a good husband, then suddenly I had nothing' ...

Mr E. is separated with four children 'it's having no one to share problems with. Being poor and seeing your children going without things that other children have'. Ms H. is separated with one child 'loneliness would be the worst — you've nobody else to confide in or share responsibility with'.[5]

The research of Evason and the CHES team, suggesting that about one third of single parents and remarried mothers experience clinically-observable symptoms of anxiety and depression, points to an iceberg of suffering. Their findings are, however, consistent with the patterns of mental illness found among other groups of women under stress. The measures used in different studies vary, so the findings from different studies are not exactly comparable. Nonetheless, it is interesting to note that Burnell and Wadsworth's and Evason's figures are similar to those of Brown and Harris, reported earlier. In Brown and Harris's sample, 31% of the working-class mothers with pre-school children were found to have symptoms of clinical depression. The figures are consistent, too, with the findings of the Waltham Forest study of children with behaviour problems. Here 39% of the mothers caring for difficult children were identified to have some degree of psychiatric disorder (Richman, Stevenson and Graham, 1982:38). Again, a study of mothers in multi-storey flats recorded 33% of the sample as depressed (Littlewood and Tinker, 1981).

Set in the context of these studies, the data from the studies of lone parents underlines the importance of material and social disadvantage. In these studies, it is the material disadvantages stemming from illegitimacy and marital breakdown which are highlighted. It is these material aspects of parenthood to which this book now returns.

NOTES

1. Townsend, P. & Davidson, N. (1982) *Inequalities in Health* (The Black Report) pp.56-7.
2. Doyal, L. (1983) 'Women's Health and the Sexual Division of Labour', *Critical Social Policy*, 7, Summer: 28.
3. Cooperstock, R. & Lennard, H. (1979) 'Some social meanings of tranquillizer use', *Sociology of Health and Illness*, Vol.1, 3, p.336.
4. Spring Rice, M. (1939) *Working class wives: their health and conditions*, p.30.
5. Evason, R. (1980: a) *Just Me and the Kids: A Study of Single Parent Families in Northern Ireland*, pp.79-80.

Part III
RESOURCES FOR FAMILY HEALTH

6 Money

6.1 INTRODUCTION

Part I described the broad patterns of family life and family health in contemporary Britain. It drew attention to the fact that, while the majority of families with children are two parent families, a significant and growing minority are headed by one (typically female) parent. These early chapters noted, too, that while most families have an income sufficient to sustain their health, an increasing minority of households with children live in poverty. Part II examined the position of families in their wider social context. It focussed on two dimensions of our social structure, describing the way in which social class and sex roles shaped an individual's experience of health. Together these two sections provide the foundation for the remainder of the book, describing the social and economic setting in which mothers work for family health. Part III examines the nature and organisation of women's health resources, while Part IV is concerned with their health responsibilities.

Potentially all household resources exert an influence on health. The tangible resources of money, housing, food, fuel and transport, like the intangible resources of time, energy and love, each play their part. The next four chapters are therefore selective. They examine resources long considered important to health (income, housing, fuel and food). They also consider one area which has received little attention in the current discussion of community care and family responsibility: transport.

In directing our attention to the home, the broader context of health can become obscured. Once described, it is all too easy to lose sight of social structure and forget that health is governed by factors beyond the orbit of the home. In an attempt to keep these wider influences in view, the following four chapters are not exclusively concerned with the allocation of resources within

families. Each chapter begins with a brief examination of the data
on the distribution of resources between families.

6.2   DISTRIBUTION OF INCOME BETWEEN
         FAMILIES

Income-production is a pre-requisite for the maintenance of a
family. Without a reliable and adequate source of income,
parents cannot provide a home for themselves and their children.
Data on this most basic health resource suggest that there are
wide differences between households.

National data on the income of households are provided by the
Family Expenditure Survey and the General Household Survey.
In 1980, the average weekly gross income of all households in
Britain, including those with and without children, was £137
(Department of Employment, 1982: a). Tables 6.1 and 6.2
describe the distribution of income which lies behind this
average. From these tables, it is possible to identify two distinct,
but not mutually exclusive, groups of low income families. One
group includes working-class households, in which the head has,
or is seeking, an unskilled manual job. An indication of their
economic position is given in Table 6.1. A second group is made
up of single parent families. The economic position of these
predominantly female-headed families is outlined in Table 6.2.
Together, the two tables provide, in a summary form, some basic
income data on the impact of social class and parental status on
family income. Although describing average differences only,
they underline the significance of these two dimensions of
Britain's social structure. Households in the top socio-economic
group command average incomes three times greater than households in the lowest group (£238 and £79 respectively). The impact
of parental status, though less profound, is still marked. The
average incomes of two parent families are twice those of one
parent families: £113 for a two parent family with one child
compared with £56 for a one parent family.

In surveying these patterns of household income, the Royal
Commission on the Distribution of Income and Wealth highlighted the importance of employment in protecting families
from poverty (Layard, Piachaud and Stewart, 1978). More
recent data confirm the fact that income falls sharply with
unemployment, and is lowest among the long-term unemployed.

Table 6.1: Socio-economic Group and Household Income:
Great Britain 1980 (number in sample = 8389)

Socio-economic group of head of household	Mean usual gross weekly income (£)*
Professional	238
Employers & managers	198
Intermediate non-manual	165
Junior non-manual	114
Skilled manual	140
Semi skilled manual & personal service	95
Unskilled manual	79
All groups	137

* based on all households

Source: adapted from OPCS (1982) *General Household Survey 1980*, Table 2.13, p. 21.

Table 6.2: Household Income in One and Two Parent Families:
United Kingdom, 1980

Household type	Average number of workers	Average number of persons	Average gross weekly income (£)
One adult, one or more children	0·8	2·90	56
One man, one woman with one child	1·7	3·00	113
One man, one woman with two children	1·8	4·00	122

Source: Department of Employment (1982) *Family Expenditure Survey 1980*, Table F, p. 17.

An analysis of data from the Family Finances Survey indicates that the unemployed are considerably poorer than those on very low wages (Bradshaw, Cooke and Godfrey, 1983:441). Part of the reason for the extremes of poverty found among unemployed families lies in Britain's social security provision for the unemployed. The unemployment benefit system introduced in 1945 was not designed to cope with long-term unemployment, with the result that insurance benefits meet the needs of the short-term unemployed only. When unemployment benefit is exhausted, families are forced to rely on means-tested supplementary benefits: the position in which around 40% of the unemployed now find themselves (ibid.:434). Further, in contrast to other categories of families dependent on supplementary benefit (like one parent families), the unemployed are the only group not entitled to the long-term rate of supplementary payment normally payable after twelve months.

While two parent unemployed families are disadvantaged within the social security system relative to one parent families, they are better placed in relation to the labour market. As the Royal Commission on the Distribution of Income and Wealth observes, 'single parent families are the most exposed, since there is only one potential earner in the family and there are children to feed' (Layard, Piachaud and Stewart, 1978:28). Not only are one parent families dependent on a solitary breadwinner, their breadwinners are predominantly women seeking employment in a segregated labour market which typically offers lower rewards to women than to men. In addition, with no deputy carer available at home, lone mothers find that their childcare responsibilities restrict their job opportunities and rates of pay more than those of their married sisters.

As a result of these barriers to employment, earnings provide a less reliable and less adequate source of income for one parent families than for couples with children. One parent families therefore rely less on earnings for their income, turning instead to the welfare state for the income necessary to maintain a home for themselves and their children. But, as we saw in Chapter 2, where income can only be secured through State benefits, poverty is a

Table 6.3: One Parent Families on Supplementary Benefit: Great Britain, December 1981

	Claimants ('000s)	Children ('000s)
All one parent families on supplementary benefit	392	666
Divorced	124	232
Separated	129	245
Single	127	169
Widowed	8	13
Prisoners' wives	4	7

Source: House of Commons Hansard, Vol. 29, 18 October 1982, cols. 69-70. Reprinted in Burghes (1982: 6), p.44.

common experience. While one parent families account for 14% of families with children, they constitute one half of the families on supplementary benefit. 392,000 one parent families were drawing supplementary benefit in 1981 (Table 6.3).

The Study Commission on the Family provides further data on the sources of income in one and two parent families (Popay, Rimmer and Rossiter, 1983:47). These data are reproduced in Table 6.4. They suggest that the majority of two parent families have earnings as their main source of income (95% in 1979). In male-headed one parent families, about 70% rely primarily on earnings. But in female-headed one parent families, the proportion drops to under a half (45%). Conversely, only a minority

Table 6.4: One and Two Parent Families by Main Source of Income: Great Britain, 1979

	State benefits	Earnings	Mainte- nance	Other items	Total no. of families with head under pension age
One parent families headed by a woman	360,000	330,000	[50,000]	[10,000]	740,000
One parent families headed by a man	[30,000]	70,000	—	—	100,000
Two parent families	270,000	5,960,000	—	[30,000]	6,260,000

Note
These broad estimates are based on a Department of Health and Social Security analysis of income and other information recorded by respondents to the 1979 family expenditure survey. They are subject to statistical error; those figures in brackets are subject to very considerable proportionate error. The figures are based on the normal employment of the head of the family, where the head is under pension age.

Source: Popay, J., Rimmer, L. and Rossiter, C. (1983) *One Parent Families,* p.47.

of two parent families (5%) depend on the State for their economic survival. Among one parent families, 30% of male-headed households and 49% of female headed housholds are in this position.

Table 6.5: Two Parent Families on Supplementary Benefit: Great Britain, December 1981

	Claimants		Children	
	Number ('000s)	%	Number ('000s)	%
Pensioners	2	1	2	—
Sick and disabled	19	5	40	5
Unemployed	370	93	821	93
All supplementary benefit	399,000*		879,000	

* the number of parents (rather than the number of claimants) on supplementary benefits is higher than this figure.

Source: HMSO and House of Commons Hansard, *Social Security Statistics 1981*, Vol. 23, 12 May 1982, cols. 277-8. Reprinted in Burghes (1982) p. 44.

Understanding the significance of data on family income is not always easy. There are four reasons, in particular, why interpretation is difficult. Firstly, the figures are always out of date, and the financial position of families is changing constantly. With the increase in unemployment, for example, the numbers of families drawing supplementary benefit is rising. The number of children on supplementary benefit because their parents are unemployed almost doubled in 1981, the latest year for which data are available. In December 1980, the figure was just under 500,000: in December 1981, it had risen to 821,000 (see Table 6.5). The Department of Health and Social Security estimate for 1983-4 puts the number of children dependent on supplementary benefit at nearly two million.

These figures on family poverty may be considered unreliable for a second reason. They provide a static picture of the financial position of one and two parent families: they do not tell us about the impact of separation and death on individual families over time. A recent study of one parent families created through divorce provides this dynamic perspective (Maclean and Eeke-laar, 1983). A national survey of 7,000 adults who were or had been divorced describes the extent of the economic deprivation which follows from marital breakdown. At the time of the divorce, fewer than one in five respondents had savings of over £500 (ibid.: 23). Reflecting this, their economic security depended less on past savings than future living arrangements. Among the custodial parents who lived alone with their children, eight out of ten lived below the poverty line. Among custodial parents who went on to form new families, through cohabitation or remarriage, three in ten were living in poverty. Separation and divorce, the authors conclude, instigate a major movement into poverty by mothers and children who, in marriage, managed to live outside it.

Maclean and Eekelaar's findings highlight a third reason for caution in the interpretation of statistics on family poverty. While they point to the poverty which results from marriage breakdown, their data describe the economic position of house-holds rather than individuals. Their data demonstrate that household income is higher among married couples with children than among lone parents with children; however, this does not mean that mothers and children necessarily enjoy a higher standard of living within marriage than outside it. As noted in Chapter 1, we have always to distinguish between the income and living standards of households, and those enjoyed by the individuals within them. A study of lone parents in Northern Ireland confirms that the majority live in poverty (around 70%). None-theless, the author found that two thirds of separated and divorced mothers in the study felt that their standard of living had not deteriorated significantly since the end of their marriage. About a quarter, in fact, felt that they were 'a bit better off' than when they were living with their husbands. Evason concludes that, 'for many of these women, single parenthood represented a movement from poverty as a result of the inequitable distribution of resources between husband and wife to poverty as a result of the lowness of benefits — not, as is popularly supposed, from adequacy to penury' (Evason, 1980: a: 22-3).

Evason's finding has been confirmed by other studies. The level of state support is low and insufficient to meet the health needs of a growing family (Piachaud, 1979, 1981). Nonetheless, for claimants whose benefit levels have been established, it is regularly paid. Moreover, for lone mothers, it is paid directly to the mother. For a majority of lone mothers, it appears that a low and reliable income over which they have control, represents an improvement in the financial arrangements which prevailed in marriage. Their income remains inadequate, but the State proves to be a more dependable partner in the struggle to maintain a family on the poverty line (Pahl, 1980). This finding has implications for the traditional way in which most benefits for two parent families are paid — through the husband. If the resources for family health are not reaching those for whom they are intended, then the method of allocation should be reviewed. Joint claims for supplementary benefit would provide one solution (Evason, 1980: a: 23).

Quantitative measures of income can provide an inadequate picture of the economic circumstances of parents and children. However, there is a specific sense in which comparisons between the incomes of one and two parent families may be invalid. This suggests a fourth reason for caution in our interpretation of data on family poverty. It has been argued that the costs of maintaining the two type of households are different: that one parent families are cheaper to run. Single parents, for example, have only one adult to feed and clothe: their weekly outgoings on these items may thus be lower. However, the Finer Committee on One Parent Families found that these savings were offset by additional expenses, particularly on food and childcare. The committee noted that fatherless or motherless families face high expenditure on food because they have less time to economise by shopping around and by home baking. They are thus forced to spend more on locally-bought convenience foods. In addition, they face child-minding costs, particularly if the parent goes out to work, including travel costs as well as any direct costs of childcare (Finer Report, 1974: 266).   '

George and Wilding similarly found that single parenthood increased, rather than reduced, family expenditure. As they note, 'motherlessness makes life more expensive' (George and Wilding, 1972: 99). Nine in ten of their fathers reported spending more since they became single parents. With no time to shop for bargains and to make things themselves, they spent more on food and clothes. They also reported spending more on 'compensating expenditure' for themselves and their children in the first year after becoming lone parents. Sweets, toys, cigarettes and drink were all cited as items bought in an attempt to compensate for their sense of loss (ibid: 100). In a more recent American study,

Chambers calculates that, deprived of the economies of scale, a mother needs over three quarters of the former family's total income to maintain the same standard of living after a separation (Chambers, 1979).

'It costs as much to run a home in terms of heating, lighting, cooking and mortgage for two of us as it did for four of us'.[1]

6.3 PATTERNS OF SPENDING WITHIN THE HOME

How much a family receives, in earnings and income-transfers, governs how much it can spend on health. A family's investment in its home and diet, and its system of heating and communication depends upon the income at its disposal. It is not surprising to find that these patterns of family expenditure closely follow those of household income. Total household expenditure among

Table 6.6: Expenditure Patterns Among Households with Children: the Impact of Income, 1981

Household with one man, one woman and two children

	Average weekly household expenditure			
	Under £120		£250 or more	
	£	%	£	%
Basic commodities				
housing	14.33	14	33.08	16
fuel, light & power	8.01	8	10.70	5
food	28.30	28	41.51	20
Other commodities				
clothing & footwear	6.68	7	15.71	8
transport & vehicles	12.19	12	32.27	15
services	6.73	7	26.84	13
alcohol & tobacco	9.62	10	11.54	6
durable household goods	7.06	7	20.57	10
other goods	7.89	8	15.80	8
miscellaneous	0.58	1	1.87	1
Total expenditure	101.39		209.90	

Source: Department of Employment (1982) *Family Expenditure Survey 1981*, Table 12, pp. 43-8.

families with children is significantly higher among the rich than the poor and among two parent families than one parent families (Department of Employment, 1982: b).

There are not only absolute differences in what families spend on health, there are relative differences as well. Poor families devote more of their household income to securing the basic commodities. The expenditure patterns among the richest and poorest households with children are described in Table 6.6. These suggest that poor households spend 50% of their income on the three health resources of housing, food and fuel. The corresponding figure for the richest households is 41%. For one parent families, over half (54%) of their weekly expenditure goes to securing the basic commodities. In two parent families (with one or more children) the figure is 44% (Table 6.7).

Statistics on family expenditure, like those on family income, deal with households and not with individuals. In so doing, the assumption is made that income is pooled and shared out in such

Table 6.7: Expenditure Patterns of One and Two Parent Households: Average Weekly Household Expenditure, United Kingdom, 1981

	One parent. with. two or more children		One man, one woman and two children	
	£	%	£	%
Basic commodities				
housing	17.51	18	22.38	15
fuel, light & power	9.03	9	8.61	6
food	25.93	27	34.42	23
Other commodities				
clothing & footwear	9.59	10	11.25	8
transport & vehicles	8.91	9	21.14	14
services	8.60	9	15.65	11
alcohol & tobacco	4.91	5	9.93	7
durable household goods	3.47	4	11.35	8
other goods/ miscellaneous	7.82	8	12.43	8
Total expenditure	95.77		147.16	

Source: Department of Employment (1982: b) *Family Expenditure Survey 1981*, Table 12, pp.43-8.

a way that all members of the house live at the same level of income. A similar assumption is made about spending: that all family members share equally in their command over resources and share equally in the benefits that these resources bring.

While this assumption is a central one, there is little empirical evidence to test and support it. As Piachaud notes, there are methodological problems about collecting material on individual income and expenditure within families (Piachaud, 1982: 470). Family finances are considered a private matter, and not a suitable topic for social investigation. Further, how much money individual members of the family receive tells us little unless we know what this income is designed to cover: all the rent and food, for example, or just cigarettes.

Nonetheless, there are studies which shed some light on income distribution in the home (Land, 1983). The OPCS survey of *Matrimonial Property*, conducted on behalf of the Law Commission, includes data on the division of responsibility for the major items of household expenditure. A significant feature of this division is that it is women who assume responsibility for meeting collective needs. In the OPCS survey, the wives typically paid for the food, fuel and rent (Table 6.8).

Table 6.8: Division of Responsibility for Household Items of Expenditure: Great Britain, 1971

Who usually dealt with	Buying food	Paying for gas/ electricity	Paying for Rent/ rates	Paying for mortgage/ rates	Dealing with any surplus
	%	%	%	%	%
Wife	89	49	61	30	36
Husband	3	38	29	59	20
Both or either	7	10	6	11	43
Other answers	1	3	4	—	1
	100=1877	100=1877	100=896 (tenants)	100=978 (owner occupiers)	100=1877

Source: Todd, J. & Jones, L. (1972) *Matrimonial Property*, OPCS, HMSO, pp. 29-30.

The findings of the OPCS survey are confirmed in other studies of housekeeping patterns. Much of this research has been concerned with poverty, describing the spending arrangements in low-income families (see Land, 1977: 166). This research suggests that it is the father who exercises most control over the income coming into the house. A certain, and usually fixed, amount of the family income is earmarked for the wife, sometimes formally identified as a housekeeping allowance (Pahl, 1980: 320). From this income, the wife pays for purchases made on behalf of the whole family, as Table 6.8 records. Using more recent data from the Family Expenditure Survey, Piachaud suggested that over 80% of the money devoted to food and over 70% of the money devoted to clothing was spent by the wife: spending on housing was not included in the analysis (Piachaud, 1982). There is also some evidence to suggest that in poor families the housekeeping money is expected to cover a wider range of items than in more affluent households (*Woman's Own*, 1975). In a study of working-class families, for example, the wife was generally found to have responsibility for all the major items of collective expenditure. Among owner-occupiers, however, the mortgage was often an item of joint expenditure (Gray, 1979).

While the wife's income is largely devoted to family purchases, her husband's income is more likely to go on items of individual expenditure. In Gray's study, for example, the husband typically paid only for his cigarettes, for visits to the pub and for the car. In addition, he was likely to share with his wife the costs of his clothing, the children's clothing, decorating and repairs, holidays and the children's pocket money (Gray, 1979: 197).

These patterns of financial responsibility reflect the patterns of domestic activity of men and women. Women tend to take responsibility for buying those items needed to perform their role: housekeeping money buys the raw materials for women's work. While this may not be an unexpected finding, it has significant implications for family health.

Firstly, the division of income between husbands and wives has implications for the way we assess living standards. It is not always valid, for example, to make inferences about family welfare directly from data on household income. In families where husbands make a contribution to items of collective expenditure or where these items are jointly purchased by husband and wife, household income may provide a reliable indication of living standards in the home. However, for many families, monies reserved by the husband for items of individual expenditure need to be deducted, since it is the residual income which provides the basic health resources of accommodation, fuel, food and clothes for the family. Thus, while gross incomes may average £122 for a two parent, two child family (1980 figures), we do not know what proportion of this figure is invested in family life. Similarly, while the rate of supplementary benefit for a two parent, two child family is £61.80 (1983 figures), we do not know how much is devoted to personal and how much to collective purchases.

The fact that women typically meet the financial costs of family life means that their income has a determining influence on living standards. Mothers' net income, rather than family gross income, may provide a more accurate measure of material well-being. In assessing living standards, therefore, we need to attend to the monies which go directly to the parent with responsibility for housekeeping. We need to examine not only housekeeping allowances, but women's earnings and child benefit. Studies suggest that these latter sources of income are particularly significant in protecting the living standards of children. Controlled by the mother, they tend to be largely committed to health expenditures. In the OPCS survey of matrimonial property, 70% of women's earnings were found to go on general housekeeping (Todd and Jones, 1972). Hunt's study of women in employment similarly noted that general housekeeping and children's clothes disposed of most of their earnings (Hunt, 1968). Studies of child benefit have found that the benefit is also an essential component of mother's income (Lister and Emett 1976; McClelland, 1982). The studies underlined the precarious, hand-to-mouth budgeting that goes on in low-income families. The payment of child benefit on Tuesday morning paid for vital resources, of food and fuel, to last the family until pay-day on Thursday night. Further, the fact that, although deducted from supplementary benefit, child benefit is still paid to the person directly responsible for the children was crucial for mothers coping with unemployment. Such evidence suggests that the shift from weekly to monthly payments for new mothers is likely to reduce the effectiveness of child benefit in protecting the living standards of children (McClelland, 1982: 5).

There is perhaps, no better mode of ascertaining what degree of comfort is enjoyed by a labourer's family, than by learning what portion of his weekly earnings he commits to his wife's disposal. It makes very material difference whether he or she holds the purse strings. That he can earn the most is granted, but she can make those earnings go the farthest.[2]

An appreciation of women's financial responsibilities is important for an understanding of family health in a second respect. Since mothers' responsibility for collective expenditure tends to consume most, if not all, the money at their disposal, their incomes need to be both regular and highly sensitive to cost changes. Incomes irregularly received or insufficiently responsive to changes in the costs of health care make it difficult for mothers to safeguard the health of their family. Stability of income, whether from state benefits, wages or housekeeping, is particularly vital for mothers coping on the poverty line. Delays in payment of supplementary benefit to a lone mother, for example, inevitably mean that her family is forced to live on an income incompatible with health: an experience for which the payment of arrears at a later date cannot compensate (Evason, 1980: a: 19). However, in times of inflation or when the family is growing, stability of income alone is not enough to protect health. When costs rise, mothers must be able to increase the amount they spend on food, fuel, clothes and housing. Yet the evidence suggests that mothers' incomes are more rigid than male earnings. Housekeeping money, for example, appears not to be index-linked, and is peculiarly unresponsive to rising prices and changing needs. (*Woman's Own*, 1975; Pahl, 1980). Similarly, supplementary benefit has been found to be insufficiently sensitive to the needs of growing children: for clothes and for school equipment as well as for food (Burghes 1980; Piachaud, 1981). The rate of child benefit, alone among the state benefits, rose more than the rate of inflation between 1979 and 1983. In 1983, it was 5p ahead of the rate of inflation.

If rising costs are not met by increased income, and debts are to be avoided, savings must be made by the housekeeper. These reductions in spending have to come, inevitably, from collective expenditure. A third major implication of the division of income within the home is therefore that savings made by the mother involve cutting consumption on items directly related to health. As the evidence reviewed in Chapters 7 and 8 indicates, mothers cut back on basic necessities in order to live within their means. Again, the consequences of such cutbacks are particularly severe for poor families, where financial solvency can often only be secured at the cost of health.

There is a fourth reason why an appreciation of housekeeping patterns is important for an understanding of family health. Worries about money are a major source of stress among lone mothers and married mothers dependent on supplementary benefit (Evason, 1980: a; Burghes, 1980). In Evason's study, it was financial worries which were most frequently reported by lone parents as the problem uppermost in their minds. Worries about money, too, have been identified as contributing to depression among mothers with children (see Chapter 5.3). Further, conflicts over money and expenditure have been identified as a major factor in marital disharmony and marital violence (Pahl, 1980; Dobash and Dobash, 1982). In such a situation, the economic inequality between husband and wife increases the wife's vulnerability to assault, and it makes it more difficult for her and her children to escape from her violent husband.

The next three chapters examine some of the collective purchases known to be most closely related to family health. They examine the data on housing and on fuel, food and transport.

NOTES

1. Lone father's evidence to the Finer Committee, published in the *Report of the Committee on One Parent Families* (1974) Cmnd. 5627, para. 5.41, p.264.
2. Eden, F. M. (1797) *The State of the Poor*, Vol. 1, p.625, quoted in Land, H. (1977) 'Inequalities in Large Families', p.166.

7 Housing and Fuel

7.1 INTRODUCTION

Income provides the raw materials for health: it buys the shelter, warmth and food that parents need to protect the welfare of their family. This chapter considers two major household purchases — accommodation and fuel — known to be closely related to child health. Like food, these are identified as items of collective expenditure. They may be bought by one family member but their benefits are seen to extend to all.

Housing and fuel consume over a quarter of net income among families with children (Department of Employment, 1982: b, Table 12). The cost of these basic resources takes a particularly heavy toll on the poor. As we noted in Chapter 6, low-income families tend to spend a higher proportion of their household income on necessities. Fuel, in particular, consumes more of the family budget among the poor than the rich. Moreover, the cost of housing and fuel has risen more sharply than the official rate of inflation indicates. In 1981, the rate of inflation was 12%. However, in that year, rents rose by 37% and fuel by 26% (Smith, 1983: 1). Because the poor spend more on essentials, their cost of living has increased more steeply than for the rest of the community.

The fact that the poor experience a higher rate of inflation than is reflected in the Retail Price Index has particularly serious consequences for families on supplementary benefit. In the six years from 1974 to 1980, supplementary benefit increased by 137%. Electricity prices, however, rose by 228% during that period. While the fuel allowance for claimants is adjusted in line with changes in the RPI, the weekly heating allowance included in the payment of supplementary benefit has been found to be inadequate to heat a family home to the minimum recommended levels (Cleaver, 1981).

In examining the resources of housing and fuel, this chapter is constrained by the data available. Where possible, it seeks out data on the material position of one and two parent families. In respect of housing, we have information from the 1970 national cohort study (Burnell and Wadsworth, 1981; 1982). Information on fuel highlights the disadvantageous position of low-income families, of which one parent families are a significant proportion. However, there appear to be almost no data which deal specifically with fuel problems and their health-effects among one parent families.

The chapter examines the patterns of housing and fuel consumption between families in Britain (sections 7.2 and 7.3). Section 7.4 considers whether there are also differences in consumption within families which result in the benefits of housing and fuel being unequally shared within the home.

7.2 HOUSING FOR FAMILIES

It is significant that, while so much interest is expressed about the home and community, relatively little attention has been paid to housing. In much of the research on the family, the home is identified as a social not a physical entity: a cluster of roles and responsibilities rather than a building of bricks and mortar.

'A woman's place is in the home' sums up many traditional views about women. Women's magazines and radio and television programmes are full of features about 'home making', but they often start from the point where the home is already provided.[1]

Good homes are seen as something which all families have, almost by definition. However, good housing is not so universally enjoyed. There are various measures of the quality of family housing, including tenure, type of accommodation and standard of amenities. Of these, it is tenure which is the commonly accepted measure of housing quality. Tenure embraces many of the other important indicators: owner occupiers, for example, generally have more security and more amenities. They are also more likely to live in a house, as opposed to a flat, and to be in a detached house rather than a terrace (OPCS, 1982: a;

Darke and Darke, 1979: 40-4). Although the standards are higher in the owner-occupied sector, the costs of housing are lower than in either public or private rented accommodation (Le Grand, 1982: 97). Moreover, it is estimated that owner-occupier households receive slightly more in housing subsidies created by the tax allowances on mortgages than council tenants receive through rent and rate allowances (ibid.: 88).

Using tenure as our indicator, we find sharp differences in the quality of housing among Britain's families. These differences follow the contours of social class. In the highest socio-economic group, the majority of families (85%) are owner-occupiers (with or without a mortgage); in the lowest group, the majority are council tenants (62%) or tenants of private landlords (11%). These patterns are described in Table 7.1.

Housing tenure is also closely related to family composition. Among two parent families, owner occupation is the most common form of tenure. One parent families are much less likely to own their own homes. Instead, most one parent families rent their homes from their local authority. Table 7.2 provides the most recent General Household Survey data which identify the housing situations of one and two parent families.

Table 7.1: Housing and Socio-economic Group: Great Britain, 1980 (Number in sample = 7542)

Socio-economic group of economically active	owner-occupied	rented: local authority / New Town	rented: private/ housing association	rented with job
Professional	% 85	3	7	5
Employers and managers	% 82	9	4	5
Intermediate non-manual	% 73	12	12	3
Junior non-manual	% 56	29	11	4
Skilled manual	% 54	36	7	2
Semi-skilled manual and personal service	% 37	49	8	5
Unskilled manual	% 28	62	11	—

Source: OPCS (1982: a) *General Household Survey 1980,* Table 3.10, p. 51.

Table 7.2: Housing Among One and Two Parent Families: Great Britain Combined Data (Number of one parent families = 1015; number of two parent families = 7878)

Family type	Tenure			
	Owner-occupied %	Rented: local authority/ New Town %	Rented: private/ housing Association %	Rented with job %
One parent families	32	56	11	2
Other families with dependent children	60	30	5	4

Source: OPCS (1980) *General Household Survey 1978*, Table 3.43, p. 50.

As in the field of income maintenance, one parent families depend heavily on the state for their housing. Over half (56%) are local authority tenants and a third (32%) are owner-occupiers: a pattern reversed for other families with dependent children. In Maclean and Eekelaar's study of the financial consequences of divorce, there was evidence of a movement between these sectors of the housing market. Those in council housing remained council tenants, while one in four owner occupiers had to leave that housing sector (Maclean and Eekelaar, 1983).

The importance of council housing for one parent families becomes more apparent when lone fathers are excluded. The CHES study of the position of five-year-olds in one parent families found striking differences in the rates of owner-occupation among male and female-headed households (Burnell and Wadsworth, 1982). Among male-headed families, 42% owned their own homes; among female-headed families, 23% were home-owners (ibid.: 31). The study also highlights the disadvantaged position of step families: home ownership was as unlikely for them as for one parent families.

The patterns of tenure described in Tables 7.1 and 7.2 underline the importance of council housing for families in poverty. As the private rented sector has shrunk in size, it is council housing which has taken on its role as the residual housing sector for the unemployed, the elderly, the sick and disabled and one parent families (Murie, 1983). Poor families have increasingly become concentrated in the public sector as more affluent families move upwards into owner occupation. Many of these poor council tenants are also welfare claimants, dependent on the state for their income as well as their accommodation. In the early seventies, just over half of the households living on supplementary benefit were council tenants and 28% were tenants of private landlords. Ten years later, in 1981, 61% of families on welfare were in council housing and 19% were in private rented accommodation. Single parent families on supplementary benefit are especially likely to be local authority tenants. Social security statistics for 1981 indicate that over three quarters of lone parents on supplementary benefit lived in council housing (Forrest and Murie, 1983: 455).

The different housing experiences of one and two parent families do not end with differences in tenure. The process by which one parent families find themselves concentrated in council housing operates to place them in the poorest public sector housing with the fewest amenities. Looking at the position of one and two parent families with council tenancies, Burnell and Wadsworth found that one parent families were twice as likely to live in a poor neighbourhood as two parent families. 'A poor neighbourhood' they identified as one 'commonly occupied by low income families where housing is closely packed together, many in a poor state of repair and properties frequently multi-occupied' (Burnell and Wadsworth, 1982: 10).

In poor neighbourhoods the standard of maintenance is likely to be low. Recent surveys have highlighted the scale of damp and disrepair in public sector housing (National Consumer Council, 1982; Family Service Units, 1983). Such problems present many dangers to health, dangers to which those families whose standards of home life depend upon the quality of council housing are most exposed.

In poor neighbourhoods the standard of household amenities is also likely to be low. As Table 7.3 describes, there are again differences in the standard of amenities enjoyed by Britain's families within as well as between tenure groups. One parent families and step families in the 1970 CHES study typically found themselves living in homes with less amenities than two parent families (Table 7.3).

Table 7.3: Proportion of Families with Adequate Household
Amenities †: Family Situation in 1975

	Two-parent family*		Step-family		One-parent family	
Owner-occupied	(97·2)	1,364	(94·8)	97	(90·6)	171
Council rented	(92·2)	783	(83·8)	167	(82·6)	379
Private rented	(58·6)	145	(52·6)	38	(57·1)	91
Percentages in brackets, N = 100%		2,482*		342		719

† This is defined as having sole use of all or sharing only one of the
following household amenities: kitchen, bathroom, indoor lavatory,
hot water supply, garden or yard.

* Representing 20% random sample

Source: Child health and education study, Burnell, I. & Wadsworth, J. (1982) 'Home Truths', *One Parent Times*, 8, p. 10.

Particularly striking is the variation in the housing standards of families
according to their tenure of accommodation. One parent families who are
council tenants, for example, are more likely to be living in homes lacking in
basic household amenities, in neighbourhoods rated as poor and experience a
greater frequency of moves than two parent families. This supports previous
suggestions that one parent families may be further disadvantaged by housing
allocation procedures and possibly the discriminative attitudes of some local
authorities.[2]

So far, this section has focussed on tenure as the indicator of
the quality of housing enjoyed by families in Britain. However,
other indicators also point to differences in the home conditions
of one and two parent families. Lone parent families are much
more likely to share their homes with other people, a fact which
makes surveys like the census an unreliable guide to the number
of lone parents in Britain. Figures from the General Household
Survey suggest that one in four (23%) single parent families are in
shared accommodation, compared with one in twenty (5%) of
married-couple families with children (OPCS, 1982: a: 22). The
CHES data suggest that one parent families are more likely to
live in flats than are two parent families (26% compared with
11%). In the sample, 18% of step families also lived in flats
(Burnell and Wadsworth, 1982). Flat-life, as noted earlier
(Chapter 5), has been found to affect adversely the mental health

of those caring for young children. In Littlewood and Tinker's study of *Families in Flats*, one third of the single mothers reported feeling isolated and lonely, and over one half reported being unduly irritable with their children (Littlewood and Tinker, 1981: 24).

Length of residence provides a further measure of housing disadvantage. The CHES study found that twice as many children in one parent families (40%) experience two or more moves in the first five years of life than do children in two parent families (20%). Housing insecurity and frequent changes of address dislocate friendship and family networks. As we have seen (Chapter 4), these networks are known to be particularly important for the welfare of one parent families, providing vital resources of company, childcare and, not infrequently, cash (Marsden, 1973; Weiss, 1979).

The starkest indicator of housing disadvantage is homelessness. In 1979, one third of all the registered homeless households were one parent families (Popay, Rimmer and Rossiter, 1983: 39). Equally disturbing is the high proportion of children from one parent families who end up in care. As noted in Chapter 2, over half of the children in care in 1979 are estimated to be children from one parent families. These grim statistics underline the fact that cohort studies and national statistics on one parent households are likely to mask the extent of housing problems facing these families. As Ferri (1976) observes, they describe 'only those who have managed to remain as a family unit in a home of their own'.

A good and secure home is essential to successful family life. There is an important sense in which this holds particularly true for one parent families, in that the presence or absence of adequate housing conditions may well tip the balance on whether such families surmount or succumb to the financial and social handicaps from which they are apt to suffer.[3]

7.3   FUEL FOR FAMILIES

Making a home involves more than paying the mortgage and paying the rent. Homes need heating and lighting if they are to provide a healthy environment for parents and children. Compared with the other basic necessities (like housing, food and clothes) fuel bills consume a relatively small proportion of the family's budget. Yet fuel bills are probably the item which present most problems for families on low incomes. Fuel bills are a major cause of debt among the poor, with the prospect of disconnection as fuel becomes too expensive to afford. In 1981, 109,000 households were disconnected from their electricity supply and there were 28,000 gas disconnections (Winfield, 1983: 9).

As these figures suggest, it is electricity bills which create special problems for low-income families. Firstly, electricity provides a more universal supply of heating and cooking than gas. Moreover, low-income households are more dependent on electricity for heating than are other households (Electricity Council, 1979: 3). Families who depend solely on electricity cannot substitute other fuels and thus spread their fuel bills. As a result, electricity-debtors are often those living in all-electric households (Berthoud, 1981: 119-20). Secondly, and reflecting the greater importance of electricity to most families, electricity bills are generally higher than gas bills. Among households with children, electricity bills are typically twice as high as gas bills (Department of Employment, 1982: b, Table 12). Higher bills are associated with more disconnections: as we noted above, nearly four times as many homes in England and Wales were disconnected for electricity debts as for gas arrears. Figures from the Policy Studies Institute indicate that electricity disconnections are concentrated among low-income families with children and with no readily available alternative source of heating, cooking and lighting. A significant proportion are single parent families.

Evason's study provides further insights into the position of lone parents. With fuel prices higher in Northern Ireland than in the rest of the United Kingdom, problems with paying the bills are perhaps not surprising. Evason found around a quarter of her sample were in debt at the time of the interview, many to more than one authority. Half of the instances of debt consisted of electricity arrears. A large proportion (nearly 50%) of the electricity debts were in excess of £300: the majority of gas debts, by contrast, were below £50 (Evason 1980: a: 27).

> *Electricity disconnections: which families are cut off?*
> 63% have children under 11
> 63% are not in stable full-time work
> 50% are unemployed
> 30% are in receipt of supplementary benefit
> 47% have no central heating
> 26% live in an all-electric home
> 16% are single parents[4]

It is possible to identify the factors which increase the vulnerability of poor families to fuel debts. The most obvious factor is the one least often recorded. Low-income families tend to spend more time at home than other families. Low-income families with children tend to be families where one or both of the parents are outside the labour market: single parent families living on supplementary benefit, two parent families with one wage earner and families with an unemployed or disabled head. Better-off families tend to be families in which the parents are out at work during the day, with their children at school or cared for outside the home (Richardson, 1977).

The now-disbanded Supplementary Benefits Commission identified other factors which increase the risks of fuel debts among poor families. They noted that 'many of the poorest people are obliged to use relatively expensive fuels (and) ... live in housing which leaves them with little choice about the type of fuel consumed' (Supplementary Benefits Commission, 1979: para. 5.14-5.15). Moreover, being poor, families with fuel debts are confined to poor housing which is difficult to heat and is without adequate insulation (Burghes, 1980: 37; Lorant, 1981: 7; Winfield, 1983: 10).

Compounding these problems of heating poor houses, is the quarterly system of payment for fuel (Supplementary Benefits Commission, 1979: para.5.14). Only 9% of households currently pay for their electricity through slot meters. For families on supplementary benefit, their electricity bill for the winter quarter constitutes, on average, 90% of their weekly income (Hutton, 1983: 9). For single parent families on supplementary benefit, the quarterly winter bill exceeds their weekly income (ibid.). The problem is, of course, greater for households in which both electricity and gas bills have to be paid within a few weeks of each other. They must save approximately two weeks income over the winter quarter to meet the cost of their fuel.

Recent changes in the payment of supplementary benefit appear to be intensifying this cycle of debt. Until 1983 the weekly supplementary benefit included an amount to cover housing expenses: rent, rates and mortgage. Under the new housing benefit scheme, local authority tenants receive their housing benefit in the form of reduced rent and rate bills and not as a cash payment. This 'rent direct' system limits the scope for budgeting on a low income. In particular, it restricts the scope of the housekeeper to shift money from one item of collective expenditure to another: using the rent allowance to temporarily shore up the fuel account for example. As a result, while the new scheme is expected to reduce rent arrears, it is anticipated that fuel debts and disconnections may rise (Hutton, 1983: 7).

Problems with fuel bills have immediate and obvious consequences for family health. Reducing consumption of gas and electricity in an attempt to save fuel leaves homes cold, and vulnerable to condensation and damp. Disconnection, in particular, brings very real health risks, risks which the Code of Practice, instituted by the Gas and Electricity Boards, is designed to minimise. A study of households without fuel described the effects that being without essential heating, lighting and cooking facilities had on the daily lives of the children and on relationships within the family. 'Depression, alcoholism, neglect, battering — the ugly faces of strain — emerged during disconnection' (Winfield, 1983: 33).

This report ... deals with the subjective experiences of ten families who lived without gas or electricity for periods ranging from 2½ weeks to two years ... As the interviewer, I have found their stories both painful and moving ... I am in awe of the strength shown by some; I am in despair at the damage done to others who may never recover from the humiliation or the feeling that they have failed their children.[5]

7.4 PATTERNS OF HOUSING AND FUEL CONSUMPTION WITHIN FAMILIES

The patterns of housing and housing disadvantage described in sections 7.2 and 7.3 affect all members of the family. However, there is evidence to suggest that housing (including fuel) affects the health of some family members more than others. Home conditions are known to influence the health and educational performance of children (Essen, Fogelman and Head, 1978: a and b). These influence, too, their risks of injury from accident. The Department of Trade's Home Accident Surveillance System, for example, suggests that the risk of a child being killed by falling from the family home is 57 times greater if the home is above first floor level than if the family live on the ground or first floor (Department of Prices and Consumer Protection, 1978). Similarly, the health of pensioners is now recognised to depend crucially on the quality of housing and heating they can afford in their old age (Tinker, 1981).

This section is concerned with these differential effects of housing and fuel on health. Understanding the observed links between housing and health is seriously hampered by lack of data on individual living standards within the home. As yet, we know relatively little about the access that different members of the family have to the scarce resources of household space, warmth and light. We know little about how heating is organised: how fuel is rationed through the day and between the rooms. However, there are clues. There are some limited data which suggest the kind of complex links between housing, caring and health. They point, firstly, to the disadvantaged position of women (and their dependents) in the housing market. They point, secondly, to the way domestic architecture structures the lives of the carers and children. They indicate, thirdly, the burden that housing and fuel bills place on family finances, and their indirect effects on the consumption of other health resources.

Firstly, women, alone and with children, are found among many of the groups officially recognised to be in special housing need (Brion and Tinker, 1980: 21). Women form the majority among the elderly, the physically disabled and the mentally disordered. Further, and more significant for us, battered women and single parents are also recognised as groups who, disadvantaged in the housing market, are in special need. Moreover, low-income families and homeless families are also recognised to have particular housing needs, and among these, female-headed families are a significant minority. The DHSS 1981 statistics on low-income families suggest that, among poor families with children, 30% are single parent households (DHSS, 1983:a). And, as recorded in section 7.2, one third of families accepted as homeless are one parent families.

Secondly, within the home, as well as within the housing market, women and children occupy a different position to that traditionally bestowed on men. The division of labour between childcare and income production is associated with a spatial separation between 'home' and 'work'. Domestic space is located away from industrial and commercial areas, a pattern associated with the expansion of residential buildings in the suburbs of towns and cities. Because caring is a domestic activity, the daily lives of young children and their mothers are based in and around the home. Chapter 4 noted that over 70% of women with pre-school children are not in paid employment: their work-time, like their leisure-time, is spent at home. Particularly important is the fact that women and their children are heavily represented among low-income families who spend more of their lives in the home. Women figure prominently among the single parents on supplementary benefit, among the non-working parents in one wage-earner families and among the carers of unemployed and disabled men.

It is thus the environment of the home which provides the conditions of work for many mothers with young children. The internal design of the home imposes very real restrictions on the way they care for their family. Small kitchens limit the possibility of cooking safely while supervising children, while play-spaces out of view of the kitchen present constant dangers to toddlers and young children.

The quality of housing determines whether the family can afford to act autonomously within their own home, or whether proximity of neighbours and the absence of private play areas dictate methods (of child-rearing) in which consideration of neighbours take priority over the interests of children ... Where there are many children, individualised treatment is ruled out if the mother is the sole domestic worker.[6]

For many families, the architecture of the home is likely to reflect social values out of line with those of its inhabitants (Brion and Tinker, 1980:7). About one third of Britain's housing is over sixty years old, built to reflect earlier ideas about the organisation of family life: for example, about the separation of cooking (and the cook) from the main activities of the family. Modern housing, however, is not necessarily easier to adapt to newer forms of living. Some modern forms, such as flats, seem particularly inflexible, imposing their own style of life on their inhabitants. This life-style seems, in many respects, to be incompatible with successful caring. The negative points about flat-life identified by a sample of mothers with young children related primarily to the caring role. Their criticisms centred on the lack of space for children, the problems of supervising their children's play, their fears about the safety of their children and the problems of access which unreliable lifts created for those living above the ground (Littlewood and Tinker, 1981:18). The children in the study had equally clear views about their homes. Flat-life was seen to structure their play activities and their social life, leaving them unable to play out and make friends.

It is not simply the externally-imposed constraints of architecture and urban design which shape the caring role and health experiences of mothers and children. There is a third respect in which housing appears to affect the home-based and home-bound more than those who work away from the house. The cost of housing and fuel is associated with a particular system of budgeting within families. There are two features of this system which have clear health-effects: the pattern of consumption and the pattern of payment. Regarding consumption, families tend to conserve their fuel during the day, saving supplies for the weekend and evening when all the family are together. Further, while the main living area may be warm at these times, bedrooms can be left unheated. A survey of housewives living on a modern housing estate noted how few families heated the living room before the evening, and most had no form of heating in the bedrooms (Adams, Ash and Littlewood, 1969). Another study found that where families had central heating, the majority switched it off when money was tight (Evason, 1980: b: 72). Such evidence suggests that the long periods of time which mothers and children spend alone in the house are not matched by high personal consumption of fuel. By contrast, during the relatively short periods when the father is at home, fuel consumption is likely to be high, and the house — or at least the living room — warm. Turning to the question of payment, again the burden tends to fall, directly or indirectly, on the person with primary responsibility for caring. As items of collective expenditure, housing and fuel are often paid for by the woman of the house (see Table 6.8). However, even where the mother is not directly responsible for fuel bills, fuel eats up income which would otherwise be available for food and other health expenditures. Changes in the system of payment for housing, as noted in section 7.3, could place further limits on the access of low-income families to an adequate diet.

In describing the role of the physical environment in family health and health care, this chapter has focussed on housing and fuel. In so doing, it has made reference to the way in which the organisation of these items is inextricably linked to that of other material resources. The next chapter examines one of these resources, looking at the patterns of food expenditure and consumption among families.

NOTES

1. Brion, M. & Tinker, A. (1980) *Women in Housing*, p.1.
2. Burnell, I. & Wadsworth, J. (1982) 'Home Truths', *One Parent Times*, 8:11.
3. *Report of the Committee on One Parent Families* (1974) (The Finer Report) Cmnd. 5629, para. 6.1, p.357.
4. Berthoud, R. (1981) *Fuel Debts and Hardship*, Policy Studies Institute, No. 601, pp.202-16.
5. Winfield, M. (1983) *The Human Cost of Fuel Disconnection*, p.1.
6. Wilson, H. & Herbert G. (1978) *Parents and Their Children in the Inner City*, p.184.

8 Food

8.1 INTRODUCTION

Food is the largest single item in the family's budget, accounting for nearly a quarter (23%) of weekly expenditure. Food consumption is closely related to social position, and is recognised to be a factor determining the health experiences of rich and poor. Food consumption has been seen to play a particularly important role in child health, with the quality of diet serving to increase or decrease a child's resistance to illness. The evidence suggests that, in childhood as in adulthood, you are what you eat, and that what you eat depends on who you are.

This chapter examines some of the material on food and family health. Section 8.2 considers the role of nutrition in the aetiology of health, while sections 8.3 and 8.4 look at the patterns of food consumption between and within families.

8.2 FOOD AND FAMILY HEALTH

Good food is associated with good health throughout the life-cycle. However, it is at the extremes of life, in infancy and in old age, that the effects of poor nutrition have been highlighted (Elbourne, 1981; Exton-Smith, 1980).

At the beginning of life, the influence of diet has been found to extend back through infancy and the pre-natal period to the health of the mother. Research into nutritional deprivation in the mid-1940s in the food-starved regions of eastern Europe has established the importance of maternal nutrition in perinatal outcome (Wynn and Wynn, 1981). Food shortages were associated with a dramatic rise in the number of low birth weight babies (babies whose birth weight is 2,500 grams or less). In

Leipzig, for example, the proportion of low birth weight babies rose from one in twenty in 1938 to one in eight in 1947 (ibid.: 8). The European food shortages correlate closely, too, with increases in the rate of congenital malformations. Again, in Leipzig, the rate climbed from a figure of 3 per 1,000 births in 1939 to 7 per 1,000 in 1947 (ibid.: 8).

The war-time food situation in Britain produced very different results. Despite overall shortages of food, food policies had the effect of reducing the unequal distribution of food between income-groups. With the supplies of meat, bread, sugar, milk, potatoes and cheese rationed, low-income families were able to improve their diet. With this improvement in diet went a sharp fall in the rates of perinatal mortality (DHSS, 1978: 12-13). Despite these advances, low birth weight and congenital malformations remain the major factors associated with infant death. The 6% of babies weighing 2,500 grams or less at birth accounted for 60% of the neonatal mortality figures (Alberman 1977: 6). Another 18% of neonatal death are due to congenital malformations (ibid.: 8).

In interpreting these patterns in Britain and eastern Europe, attention has focussed on the nutritional status of mothers before and at the time of conception. It was the sudden deterioration in the mother's food supply in the weeks before and after conception that was associated with the sharp rise in the number of low birth weight and malformed babies born in Germany and Poland in the aftermath of World War Two. A process of transmitted nutritional deprivation has also been identified in the British data. However, Baird suggests that it is the nutritional status of the mother not only at conception, but one generation earlier at the time of her own birth, which is critical (Baird, 1972: 323). The data linking spina bifida with vitamin deficiency around the time of conception has further fuelled concern about the role of nutrition in foetal development (Smithells et al., 1980).

The factor most closely related to mortality and to later morbidity is the weight of the baby at birth. The ultimate weight of a baby is determined by the length of gestation and by its growth rate in the uterus. Both of these are affected by socio-economic factors, but growth rate more than length of gestation. Again, the effects may be fairly direct, as when growth rate is reduced secondary to maternal nutrition; or they may be indirect, as when a mother herself, stunted by malnutrition at adolescence, is unable to support normal growth-rate in her own infant. Another indirect effect is through maternal infection in pregnancy, more common in conditions of poverty, which may reduce both length of gestation and growth rate.[1]

Table 8.1: Birthweight, Social Class and Marital Status (1970)

	Mean length of gestation (weeks)	Mean birth Weight: (grams)	% of babies born 2,500 grams or less
Social class			
1 & 2	40·20	3,377	4·5
3	40·19	3,356	5·6
4 & 5	40·05	3,264	8·2
Unsupported mothers: single, separated and divorced	39·86	3,171	9·5

Source: Chamberlain, R. et al. (1975) *British Births 1970, Vol. 1, The First Week of Life*, Tables 3.12 and 3.3, pp. 81 and 85.

Birthweight correlates closely with both social class and marital status. Data from the 1970 British Births Survey demonstrate the steady decline in mean birth weight through the social classes. Among babies born to unsupported mothers, who have no official class allegiance, mean birth weights are the lowest of all. The percentage of low birth weight babies born to single, separated and divorced women is twice that found among the babies born into social classes one and two (Chamberlain et al., 1975:85). These data are described in Table 8.1.

The effects of nutrition are not, of course, limited to infancy. The health of pre-school and school-aged children also depends on the quality of their diet. Again, research into the impact of food shortages in eastern Europe in the late forties demonstrated that dietary deficiency depresses growth (Howe and Schiller, 1952). Contemporary studies in Britain are hampered by the fact that poor nutrition is likely to be part of a complex of social disadvantage, with the result that it is difficult to separate the effects of nutritional deprivation from those of wider social deprivation (Blaxter, 1981:128). Although chronic malnutrition is no longer considered to exist among Britain's children, there is evidence to suggest that some families are considerably better fed than others. This evidence is considered in the section which follows.

8.3 HOUSEHOLD PATTERNS OF FOOD CONSUMPTION

Like other health resources, food expenditure is linked to household income and household composition. Data from the *Family Expenditure Survey* indicate that a high-income family with two

Table 8.2: Spending on Main Food Items in Families With Children: Great Britain, 1981

(A) *Household income*	One man, one woman and two children: gross normal weekly income of household	
	Under £120	£250 or more
	£	£
Milk	2.61	3.15
Poultry and undefined meat	2.36	2.92
Beef, veal, mutton, lamb	2.11	4.05
Bread	1.61	1.54
Vegetables (not potatoes)	1.59	2.02
Biscuits and cakes	1.42	1.96
Potatoes	1.21	1.18
Fruit	1.09	2.07
Sweets and chocolates	0.92	1.25
Total food expenditure	28.30	41.51

(B) *Household composition*	One adult, two or more children	One man, one woman and two children
	£	£
Milk	2.23	2.86
Poultry and undefined meat	2.16	2.74
Beef, veal, mutton, lamb	1.75	2.75
Bread	1.42	1.63
Vegetables (not potatoes)	1.54	1.78
Biscuits and cakes	1.38	1.83
Potatoes	1.23	1.26
Fruit	1.15	1.53
Sweets and chocolates	0.77	1.10
Total food expenditure	25.93	34.42

Source: Department of Employment (1982: b) *Family Expenditure Survey, 1981,* Table 12, pp. 43-4.

parents and two children spend one and a half times as much on food as an equivalent low-income family (see Table 8.2). High-income families spend twice as much on fresh fruit and carcass meat as poor families, but less on the 'filler' foods of bread and potatoes. Household composition, similarly, is related to spending on food (see Table 8.2). One parent families spend less on food than two parent families, with particularly sharp differences in expenditure on meat, poultry and fresh fruit. Interestingly, it is two parent families and high-income families who spend most on sweets and chocolates.

Associated with these patterns of household expenditure, are income-related patterns of food consumption. Table 8.3, drawn from the national survey of *Household Food Consumption and Expenditure*, provides details of individual consumption of selected food items (in ounces per week). Average individual consumption of 'good food' — particularly of meat, and fresh fruit and vegetables — is significantly higher in high-income households. Conversely, individual consumption of carbohydrates is significantly lower, with low-income families eating

Table 8.3: Household Income and Individual Food Consumption: oz per person per week: Great Britain, 1980

	Gross weekly income of head of household	
	£67-£110	Over £250
Milk	4	4
Cheese	4	5
Beef, veal, mutton, lamb & pork	16	23
Poultry and other meat products	20	17
Fresh vegetables (not potatoes)	27	36
Fresh fruit	18	32
White bread	24	12
Potatoes	45	36
Sugar	12	8

Source: Ministry of Agriculture, Fisheries and Food (1982) *Household Food Consumption and Expenditure: 1980*, Table 20, pp. 104-106.

twice as much white bread per head as high-income families.

The data contained in Table 8.3 suggest that poorer families tend to have diets higher in calories than more affluent households. Although higher in bulk, these diets are generally recognised to be lower in quality.

Obesity is known to have increased in Britain since the 1940s among both adults and children. There has been a dramatic change since the early years of the century, when the poor suffered from malnutrition and obesity was a problem only for the rich. Now obesity is more of a problem for working class people — two out of every five working class women are seriously at risk because they are overweight.[2]

While income has a decisive impact on individual food consumption, the impact of household composition appears to be more muted. As Table 8.4 shows, average individual consumption does not vary in a consistent way betwen one and two parent families. However, there is evidence that large families, with three or more children, have poorer diets than other families. Their

Table 8.4: Household Composition and Individual Food Consumption: oz per person per week: Great Britain, 1980

	One adult, one or more children (ozs)	Two adults, one child (ozs)	Two adults, two children (ozs)
Milk	4	4	4
Cheese	3	4	4
Beef, veal, mutton, lamb and pork	11	18	13
Poultry and other meat products	20	20	18
Fresh vegetables	21	26	22
Fresh fruit	17	21	19
White bread	23	22	20
Potatoes	37	41	39
Sugar	12	10	9

Source: Ministry of Agriculture, Fisheries and Food (1982), *Household Food Consumption and Expenditure: 1980*, Table 23, pp. 114-116.

average intake of iron and energy is below that recommended by the DHSS and is declining (Roll, 1983:10).

The *Family Expenditure Survey* and the survey of *Household Food Consumption and Expenditure* derive their statistics from data on households. Individual food consumption is calculated from household data, on the assumption that the food in the weekly shopping basket is equally divided among the family. As in other areas of family life, such an assumption is not always valid. Instead, the distribution of food within the home is governed by perceptions of need and responsibility. These perceptions are explored in the next section.

8.4   DISTRIBUTION OF FOOD WITHIN THE FAMILY

Household data suggest that low-income families and one parent families spend less in absolute terms but more in relative terms on food than high-income families (see Tables 6.6 and 6.7). The diets of poor families are also proportionally higher in carbohydrates and lower in meat, cheese, fruit and vegetables (see Tables 8.2, 8.3). Behind such general tendencies, there are more subtle processes at work. These processes make the purchase, preparation and serving of food a highly symbolic activity. In the provision and consumption of meals, we can see outlined the complex division of responsibilities and resources which govern the home. In looking at family food, we are therefore looking in a very direct way at the organisation of family life.

The preparation and serving of food holds a special and deeply significant place in all societies. Obviously food sustains social life in a very literal sense: without it, we would die. But food is also an expression of social relationships. In most cultures, food is an indicator of social worth: the best food is reserved for the most privileged members of the household, while those who serve make do on less and worse. More generally, food is seen to reflect the quality of the institution in which it is prepared. In our culture, good homes are places where, among other things, there is good home cooking (Murcott, 1982:a:80).

The significance of food in social relationships has become a recent focus of interest. Particularly relevant are two studies of family food, conducted recently in South Wales and York (Murcott, 1982:a, b, 1983; Kerr and Charles 1982, 1983). These studies suggest that meal times are important because they are family times: eating is an example of what families do together. However, their significance extends further. Meals and meal times also reflect roles within the family. The organisation of cooking and eating marks out the roles of husband and wife, and parent and child.

In most housholds it is women who cook. In Murcott's study in South Wales, men helped out and lent a hand or sometimes cooked 'things on toast' but women remained in charge of the day-to-day purchasing and preparation of food (Murcott, 1982: b:691). In many homes, these responsibilities lie at the heart of women's caring role: being the housekeeper means, first and foremost, ensuring that the family is well fed. Although pivotal, cooking is not altogether typical of women's caring activities. Unlike housework and childcare, cooking is capital-intensive. As we have seen, cooking consumes nearly one quarter of weekly household income in the average two-parent, two-child family. By contrast, cleaning and childcare are more labour intensive: they demand time and energy, but not much money. Food thus occupies a unique place in the domestic economy; touching on both the division of labour and the division of income within the home. As a result, cooking becomes a mark of the housewife's skill as a cook and as a housekeeper. Her competence in the kitchen rests on her being able to cook well and spend her money wisely.

In a number of important ways, cooking and eating is about the exercise of control within the family. Because of its pivotal place in the division of labour, food is an arena in which women seek to control the family budget. Its pivotal position, too, makes cooking and eating a highly effective means of controlling the behaviour of adults and children. However, the question of who controls whom is by no means straightforward. Parents use eating to punish and reward their children: children, in turn, offer and refuse their co-operation at meal times in a family battle of wills (Eppright et al., 1969; Lawrence, 1979). Food, too, enters into marital relationships, with both wives and husbands known to be highly sensitive about what is cooked and eaten (Murcott, 1982:a).

This section now looks at two areas in this complex political economy of family life. It examines the financial implications of food expenditure for the household budget and the social implications of food preparation for family relationships.

(a) Food and Family Finances

Food occupies a key role in the domestic economy of poor families. Of all the basic necessities, spending on food is the one over which the housewife can exercise most control. Housing and, to a lesser extent, fuel, are fixed items on the household budget, offering little opportunity for economy. Families on low incomes, therefore, turn to their food budget in an attempt to make ends meet (Burghes, 1980:30; Evason, 1980:a:25). It is through their diet that families confront and try to contain their poverty, designing diets which enable them to live within their incomes. As one separated mother explained 'You can always make the food stretch, but you can't cut down the price of clothes' (Evason, 1980:a:83). It is thus at meal times that the meaning of poverty is most acutely felt.

A series of surveys have recorded the diets of families on the poverty line (Boyd Orr, 1937; Rowntree, 1941; Marsden, 1973). The results from one recent survey of sixty-five families on supplementary benefit are reproduced in Table 8.5. The chart illustrates a number of features of meal times among the poor. Firstly, the diet sheets indicate that collective consumption is low. Meals at home are often missed, and those that are served are invariably one-course affairs. Moreover, the diets are monotonous and lack the nutritional balance recognised as necessary for long-term health. Carbohydrates figure prominently: toast, bread, chips and spaghetti are staple items for both parents and children. Primary protein is limited to eggs and sausages, although fish and fish fingers are included in some families' diets. Fruit does not feature in any form, fresh, tinned or frozen, and vegetables appear only in the guise of egg salad.

The diet sheets bring out a second common feature of meal times on the poverty line. While the collective consumption of food is low, there are generational differences in eating patterns. Parents in the survey noted how they went without to leave enough food for their children. Reflecting this, the children were generally better and more regularly fed than their parents. One in seven of the children (15%) had less than three meals during the previous twenty-four hours. Three out of four of the parents had less than three meals during this period: one half had two meals and one quarter only one.

Table 8.5: Meal Times on Supplementary Benefit: Meals Eaten by a Sample of Parents and Their Children on the Day of or the Day Before the Interview: England and Scotland, 1980

Adults' Meals

Breakfast	*Lunch*	*Tea*	*Supper*
Nothing	Toast, coffee	Rice and fish	Milk, biscuits
Nothing	Fish & chips	Nothing	Nothing
Tea	Nothing	*Mother:* Sandwich; *Father* Sausage, egg & chips	*Father:* Boiled egg & tea
Drink	Soup	Drink	Drink
Nothing	Nothing	Nothing	Egg salad
Coffee	Nothing	Spaghetti	Tea
Nothing	Egg & toast	Nothing	Nothing
Tea & toast	Tea & biscuit	Tea & toast	Nothing

Children's Meals

Breakfast	*Lunch*	*Tea*	*Supper*
Cereal, egg, toast	School dinner or sausage and beans	Rice and fish	Hot chocolate, biscuits
Cereal	Pie & chips	Nothing	Bread & butter
Toast & tea	School dinner or soup & yogurt	Sausage, egg & chips	Toast & tea
Cereal & toast	Fish fingers & potatoes	Soup	Beans on toast
Cereal	School dinner	Nothing	Egg salad
Cereal	School dinner	Spaghetti	Tea & sandwich
Cereal	Beans on toast	Sausage & chips	Nothing
Cereal	School dinner	Fish fingers, sausage & beans	Orange juice

Source: Burghes, L. (1980) *Living from Hand to Mouth: A Study of 65 Families Living on Supplementary Benefit*, Table 7, p.34.

Thirdly, Table 8.5 suggests that school meals are an important item in the diet of children in poverty. Marsden noted in his study of fatherless families dependent on supplementary benefits that school meals were the staple diet for one third of the children (1973:44). Finding the money to feed the children during the weekends and during school holidays was often difficult, with families running into debt and sending their children to eat with friends and relatives (ibid.:45). This study, like Burghes' study, was conducted before the 1980 Education Act removed the controls on local authorities governing the price and nutritional standards of school meals. As a result, school meals now cost more: the average price rose from 35p in 1979 to 50p in 1982, an increase of 40%. The proportion of children taking school meals correspondingly dropped over that period, from two-thirds to one half (Roll, 1983: 112). While children on supplementary benefit and family income supplement are still entitled to free school meals, the legal entitlement no longer extends to other children in low-income households. Moreover, it is now more difficult to know what poor children are eating at school and what nutritional benefit they are deriving from their meals.

The diet sheet indicates a fourth feature of the eating patterns of poor families. As well as the generational differences in food consumption recorded in Table 8.5, there is evidence of sexual differences as well. On two occasions, the mother and father are described as having different meals. The fact that family meal times can contain different diets for men and women (and for adults and children) has been noted in other studies (Oren, 1974). As part of her role as the provider of food, it is the mother's responsibility to ensure that her husband and her children are well fed. Seeing the children go without food is thus especially upsetting and especially guilt-provoking for women in poor families: 'the children get hungry and cross and I feel guilty' (Burghes, 1980:32).

It is not only in two parent families that mothers tend to bear the burden of sacrifice. Studies of one parent families suggest that here, too, mothers go short to protect the diet of their children. Marsden, in his study of 116 lone mothers, noted how they hoarded food for their children, cutting down and doing without to provide them with a full dinner. He noted, too, a stress reaction to living on a low income, in which the carers economised on their own food more than the size of their income dictated (Marsden,

1973:43). However, cutting their own consumption did not always mean getting thin. Poor diets were also associated with obesity (ibid.:42). Similarly, Evason's survey of 700 lone parents found that food was the item on which economies were most likely to be made, and invariably they were achieved by the mother going short herself (Evason, 1980:a:25).

A separated wife said, 'in the school holidays I sometimes stand there and cook a full dinner for them and tell them to go in the kitchen and get it and when they say, "where's yours?", I say I'm on a diet'. Another woman said, 'I'd rather the children had the food than I did. It seems to satisfy me more. *They* don't go short, I do' ... A separated wife recalled, 'it's like the old saying, "in a poor family, the wife gets nowt"'.[3]

An appreciation of the woman's role in food production leads us to the second area in which food features in the political economy of the family. There is considerable evidence to suggest that food, in the form of meals and snacks, is used to express desired and valued patterns of behaviour and to control those who step out of line.

(b)   Food and Family Relationships
Within the limits of their income, the food that families eat reflects their views about what constitutes the right food for families. As the shoppers and the cooks, it is women who are most involved in and committed to providing the best for their family. The Newsoms, for example, in their study of Notting-hamshire families in the 1950s, recorded the care which mothers took over selecting their babies' diets and the knowledge mothers had about the food preferences and food foibles of their children; they described, too, the care that mothers took in preparing meals for their children and their concern when they didn't eat them (Newsom and Newsom, 1970: 216-56). The authors note, in particular, the mothers' concern that their children have 'proper' meals, and avoid filling up on sweets and snacks (ibid.: 223).

The more recent studies, conducted in Wales and England, confirm that mothers have clear ideas about what their children, and their partners, should be eating (Murcott, 1982:a; Kerr and Charles, 1983). Again, among these respondents, particular significance is attached to them having a cooked dinner: a decision often resulting in the mother's food preferences becoming eclipsed and her patterns of spending on food distorted by hefty bills for meat.

Essentially, a cooked dinner is composed of meat, potatoes and at least one additional vegetable and gravy. So described it is immediately recognisable to anyone remotely acquainted with British eating. While reducible to a familiar cliché, it connotes a great deal more. For a cooked dinner is regarded as a 'proper' meal par excellence. As such, women who took part in the study, believe it is necessary to the health and welfare of their household. They have no 'worries' about their family's diet, 'as long as they are getting their dinners'. It is a meal to come home to after work or school. And, often as not, a cooked dinner is instanced as especially enjoyable, everyone's favourite.[4]

A cooked dinner is seen to constitute a proper meal. Correctly served, it consists of 'proper' meat and 'real' vegetables. Sausages and baked beans do not qualify on either score, while chops and peas do. The Sunday dinner epitomises proper eating, for both children and adults; in many families it may be the only occasion on which they eat fresh vegetables (Kerr and Charles, 1983:11). The Sunday dinner and Sunday tea can have a determining influence on the eating patterns for the rest of the week, consuming a large proportion of the family's food budget in one day. Kerr and Charles noted in their survey of mothers in York that, in eating properly on Sunday, some families found themselves forced to eat badly (in their terms) through the week. The cost of meat, in particular, can force families to make cuts in their consumption of other foods: in fruit and fresh vegetables for example.

Such findings are particularly significant in the context of the earlier discussion of poverty. Proper meals appear beyond the means of families on supplementary benefit (see Table 8.5). Sundays, like weekdays, are days when the family cannot join in and celebrate the British tradition of a cooked dinner, which appears to be so central to popular ideas about family life.

In explaining the patterns of family food, two themes have been stressed in the recent studies. Firstly, it is suggested that cooked dinners and proper meals mark out the boundaries of healthy eating. Proper eating ensures a well-balanced diet. While proper meals are healthy meals, there are health-promoting foods which are not universally regarded as proper foods. In the study of families in York, for example, mothers recognised that salads were good for you. However, they were not always regarded as a suitable substitute for a cooked dinner. Social class was a factor, with mothers (and their partners) on higher incomes being more ready to incorporate salads into the family diet (Kerr and Charles, 1983:2).

Secondly, the particular food preferences of fathers and children have been found to play a major role in shaping the patterns of household eating. Women report that, in general terms, they cook the proper meals that their families like (Newsom and Newsom, 1970:233). An early American study of 2,000 households found that the food preferences of fathers are the strongest influence on family meal planning (Eppright et al.:1969). More recently, Kerr and Charles, in their study of York households, similarly found that the partner's preferences are often decisive, with the result that menus are more traditional than the woman would choose to cook for herself and her children (Kerr and Charles, 1983:15). Moreover, the meals tend to be more elaborate and time-consuming; they are more expensive too. Her partner's food preferences can also overrule the mother's commitment to healthy food. Chips and grills, for example, may figure strongly in the family diet for this reason (ibid.:16). Changing the family eating habits involves challenging many deeply-held assumptions about the woman's role as the server of food. The fact that arguments over diet and food preparation figure strongly in accounts of marital violence suggests that women's conservatism may indeed have a material basis. A number of women in the study by Dobash and Dobash mentioned that arguments about food provided the trigger for violence. One respondent, describing the typical build-up to an assault recounted 'he would say ... "There's never anything but bloody cheese, cheese, cheese, cheese all the time"' (Dobash and Dobash, 1982:191).

Children, as well as husbands, are influential in shaping the family diet. Studies suggest that children exercise less direct control over the family meals than their fathers: in general terms, it appears that children get what they are given. However, in choosing meals for the children, mothers tend to select foods they will eat, often from the fairly limited range of 'children's' foods: fish fingers, beefburgers, baked beans and chips (Kerr and Charles, 1983:36). Moreover, the York study found that where one child was particularly choosy, the diet of all the children would be restricted to the few foods they all would eat. It is important to note, however, that diets restricted to fish fingers and baked beans result not only from consumer preferences: as we have seen, poor families rely on these convenience foods, as items which are relatively cheap both to buy and to cook.

Biscuits, cakes and chocolates are beyond the means of families on the poverty line (see Table 8.5). Above the poverty line, it is estimated that one fifth of all food and drink is taken between meals (Lang, 1983:14). Data suggest that sweets, biscuits and cakes are crucial to the well-being of many families (Eppright et al.: 1969; Kerr and Charles, 1983). Their health-giving properties are not nutritional ones, however. They provide what George and Wilding (1972) describe as 'compensating expenditure' to help cope with stress. More specifically, they provide a quick and convenient way of keeping children in order. Eppright et al. (1969), in their American study, found that one quarter of the mothers used food, and sweets in particular, as a reward for good behaviour. As Kerr and Charles note, sweets are the most instant of instant foods and can be served more quickly than fruit which often has to be peeled and cut for young children. They are cheaper and, most important of all, more popular. When going about the business of caring — washing, cleaning, travelling, shopping — children often become bored, noisy and irritable. Sweets and biscuits are treats which can help women cope with their caring duties and their children at the same time. As we have seen, the task of reconciling these responsibilities is more difficult for familes where housing is poor and money is in short supply. Yet, significantly, more is spent on treats in more affluent households where material deprivations are not so acute (see Table 8.2).

Treats play a particularly crucial role in the management of children in public places: on the street, on buses and in shops. The next chapter turns to the question of the family's access to these public facilities. It examines transport as a resource for health.

NOTES

1. Alberman, E. (1977) 'Facts and Figures' in Chard T. and Richards, M. (eds.) *Benefits and Hazards of the New Obstetrics*, p.4.

2. Politics of Health Group (1980) *Food and Profit*, p.4.
3. Marsden, D. (1973) *Mothers Alone*, p.44.
4. Murcott, A. (1982: b) 'On the social significance of the "cooked dinner" in South Wales', *Social Science Information*, Vol.21, 4-5: 21-2.

9 Transport

9.1 INTRODUCTION

This chapter examines a major item of household expenditure not traditionally included in discussions of health. While income, housing and diet have all been cited in the aetiology of health, little attention has been paid to transport. Yet a family's access to shops, play-spaces and medical services depends upon the availability of a reliable and speedy means of travel. Employment opportunities, too, require an efficient transport system if parents are to be able to secure jobs commensurate with their training and qualifications.

This chapter explores some aspects of travel and transport for family health. It is divided into three sections. These are concerned respectively with the geography of family life and the patterns of transport between and within households with children.

9.2 THE CHANGING GEOGRAPHY OF FAMILY LIFE

There are marked differences in the extent to which families make use of the resources available in the community. As we observed in Chapter 3, there is an Inverse Care Law in the pattern of medical utilisation, with working-class households and ethnic minority families making less use of health services than their need for care would indicate. The question of under-utilisation has generally been discussed in terms of the personal characteristics of the potential patients. It is suggested, for example, that they hold traditional attitudes both to illness-causation and lay care which inhibit their take-up of professional services (Pill and Stott, 1982; McKinlay, 1973). More recently, however, attention has shifted away from the client, towards the structure of the service. The question of under-utilisation is increasingly seen as one which includes the organisation and delivery of medical care. Studies have highlighted, for example, the style of communication often found within GP's surgeries, hospitals and antenatal clinics. Patients have been found to spend long periods of time in crowded waiting areas for the attention of professionals, who dispense their care with little exchange of words (Cartwright and O'Brien, 1976; Graham and McKee, 1980). Important, too, is the geography of modern medical care, with its increasingly centralised provision of services to larger and more diffuse communities. The decline in home visits by general practitioners and the development of health centres to replace single-handed practices has meant longer journeys for patients wanting to see their doctor. Similarly, the expansion of child health clinics and the concomitant reduction in the domiciliary visits of health visitors to families with young children has increased the time and money that families invest in reaching the service. The centralisation of casualty departments, closing down local units and transferring their facilities to district hospitals, is also anticipated to have the effect of distancing families from those responsible for their care (Calnan, Abson and Butler, 1982). Working-class families in particular are likely to have further to travel, as the communities in which they live tend to be poorly provided with medical services (Backett, 1977:111).

This changing geography of medical care is repeated in the patterns for the marketing of food (Department of Industry, 1975). The increasing concentration of food retailing in fewer, larger shops has necessitated a policy of few-and-far-between, with the growth of chain-store shopping areas drawing on large catchment areas. With the consequent demise of local shopping precincts and corner shops, families have to travel further and pay more to find a comprehensive range of fresh foods at competitive prices. In a study of shopping behaviour in Oxford, only one in five of those responsible for the household grocery purchases lived within walking distance of a supermarket (Bowlby:1978). As a result, most of the housewives in the study relied on local small businesses for their grocery provisions.

The spatial organisation of shops and public services has particular implications for children and those who care for them. Like the elderly, children and their carers are heavily dependent on quick and easy access to resources outside the home. Access is particularly important in times of emergency. Children are known to be more at risk of accidental injury than any other group in the community. The major hazards — road accidents, falls, burns, poisonings — all require speedy medical attention. An efficient mode of transport is essential, too, if parents are to survive the emotional stresses associated with caring for young children: play groups, and drop-in centres for mothers and toddlers, for example, can be lifelines only to those able to reach them in time.

Access to services does not rely wholly upon transport, of course. Telephones offer a rapid means of communication, by which carers can make contact with the outside world without leaving the house. Like other resources, the possession of telephones is unevenly distributed through the population. Families without telephones are often those short of the basic resources for health. As Table 9.1 describes, it is among low-income households and one parent families that fewest telephones are found.

Table 9.1: Households With Telephones

Household income and household composition	*Percentage with a telephone*
Household income:	
under £120 a week	60
£250 or more a week	95
Household composition:	
one adult, one or more children	64
one man, one woman, two children	85
All households	76

Source: Department of Employment (1982: b) adapted from *Family Expenditure Survey 1981*, Table 4, p. 7.

Households without telephones tend also to be households without alternative means of communication. Specifically, they tend to be households without cars. It is the availability of private transport which is the focus of the following section.

9.3 PATTERNS OF TRANSPORT AMONG FAMILIES

The last thirty years have seen a major change in passenger transport in Britain. Most noticeable has been the increase in household car ownership. In 1953, there were 57 cars per 1,000 population; in 1979, there were 272 (Central Statistical Office, 1981:161). With the growth of private transport has come the decline of public transport. The use of buses and coaches, in particular, has fallen over the last three decades (Goodwin, 1982). These trends are outlined in Figure 9.1.

While car-ownership has risen sharply, it has not increased uniformly across the population. Like other consumer durables, cars are a measure of social and economic advantage. Car ownership thus follows the distribution of income. In social class one, than nine in ten households have at least one car, and one in three have two or more cars. In social class five, three in ten have a car (see Table 9.2). Reflecting these patterns, the use of public transport is also class-related. Trains, both underground

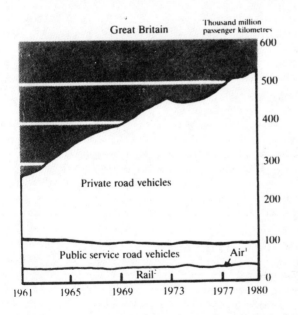

Figure 9.1:
Passenger
Transport Use

1 Domestic scheduled journeys only including Northern Ireland and the Channel Isles.
2 British Rail plus London Transport only: for the years shown, through journeys were double counted. Means of estimating season tickets were revised in 1962 and 1975.
Source: Central Statistical Office (1981) *Social Trends 1982*, Table 9.2, p. 159.

and overground, are more heavily used by middle-class travellers. Buses and coaches, however, are a predominantly working-class mode of transport. A National Consumer Council Survey of travel users found the highest rates of bus-use among those on the lowest incomes (see Table 9.3).

Car ownership is a measure which also marks out one parent and two parent families. Over 80% of two parent families own a

Table 9.2: Households With Cars: Distribution by Social Class: Great Britain, 1980

Socio-economic group of economically active heads of household (percentages)	Number of cars or vans available to households			
	None	1	2	3 +
Professional	9	55	29	7
Employers and managers	6	50	36	8
Intermediate non-manual	18	63	16	3
Junior non-manual	36	50	12	2
Skilled manual	25	59	14	2
Semi-skilled manual	49	43	7	1
Unskilled manual	71	27	2	—

Source: Central Statistical Office (1981) *Social Trends 12: 1982,* Table 9.3, p. 160.

Table 9.3: A Social Class Profile of Public Transport Users: United Kingdom 1979-80

Proportion of each group who had travelled by bus in the previous month	%
Professional/managerial	35
Clerical	46
Skilled manual	51
Partly or unskilled manual	57
Lowest income group	63
Whole sample	50

Source: Potter, J. (1982) *Public Transport,* Consumer Concerns Survey Special Paper 6, National Consumer Council, p. 7.

Table 9.4: Households With Cars: The Impact of Family
Structure, 1981

Household composition (percentages)	Number of cars or vans available to household			
	None	1	2	3 +
One adult, one or more children	68	30	2	—
One man, one woman, one child	21	60	18	1
One man, one woman, two children	18	61	20	1

Source: Department of Employment (1982: b) *Family Expenditure Survey*, Table 4, p. 7.

car; among one parent families, the proportion drops to just over 30% (see Table 9.4).

The statistic contained in Tables 9.2 and 9.4 indicate, in general terms, the proportion of British households with a car. However, as in other areas of family life, data on households are not a reliable guide to the living standards of individuals. As the section below suggests, access to transport is not always equitably distributed within households.

9.4   PATTERNS OF TRANSPORT WITHIN FAMILIES

The majority of households in Britain have the use of a car or van. The General Household Survey suggests that the figure now is 65%. However, such a figure tends to overestimate the proportion of the population who have access to the family car. Firstly, not all car-owning adults have a licence. Despite the sharp increase in car ownership over the last twenty years, the proportion of men holding driving licences is twice that of women. In the mid-1970s, 70% of men but only 30% of women held driving licences (Department of Transport: 1979). The proportions are similar among housewives and women in employment, although among the younger age groups licence holding is increasing faster for women than for men.

Secondly, access to the family car depends on the patterns of use of other members of the household. Studies suggest that men have first claim to the car, for travel to and from work. Women's access to the car thus correlates closely with their husbands' mode of travel to work (Hillman, Henderson and Whalley, 1974).

Bowlby's study in Oxford, mentioned earlier, found that although 62% of housewives lived in households owning at least one car, only half of this group had a car available during the day (Bowlby, 1978). With the car unavailable during normal working hours, women tend to find their access restricted to evenings and weekends (Pickup, 1981:8). Only in households with two cars, are women found to have equal access to car-transport.

Because of this system of distribution, sex differences in mobility and travel patterns tend to override those of car-ownership. Women, in households both with and without a car, have a lower geographical mobility than men. Associated with this lower mobility are distinctive patterns of travel among women in the labour market and in the community. These patterns involve women in more 'pedestrian exposure' than men: they cross more roads and walk farther each day than men (Todd and Walker, 1980). The quality of pavements and footpaths and the safety of pedestrian crossings are therefore particularly important for women and the children who accompany them.

Among women in the labour market, domestic responsibilities and low mobility shape their travel and employment patterns. Women workers tend to rely on slower and less reliable modes of transport than men. They rely more on public transport. The 1975 National Travel Survey found that, in London, over half the women in full-time employment used public transport compared with only one third of male workers. Walking, too, is a predominantly female mode of transport, particularly for part-time workers. In London, 16% of full-time women workers and 38% of the part-timers walked to work: the figure for all men workers was 8% (Department of Transport, 1979).

Associated with these travel patterns, women tend to work closer to home than men. In the National Travel Survey, men were found to travel nearly twice as far to work as women (10.4 km compared to 5.8 km for the average work journey length). Other studies confirm these patterns. They suggest that women rely more on local employment opportunities than men. Because women depend on slower modes of transport and because travel costs comprise a larger proportion of women's income than men, accessibility of work is a key factor determining whether women join the labour market (Klein, 1974).

Proximity and accessibility also figure strongly in the activity patterns of women in the community. Like women in employment, women at home with children do most of their travelling during normal working hours. These are the hours when shops, schools and play-groups are open, when children's walks are scheduled and visits to the clinic are arranged. The social life of housewives with children, too, takes place during the day (Pickup, 1981:2).

The daily responsibilities of childcare and housekeeping involve frequent journeys to and from the home. The National Travel Survey, for example, found that housewives make twice as many shopping journeys as the average for all adults aged between 21 and 64. They also make three times as many escort journeys. Most of these involve travelling to and from their children's school (Pickup, 1981:4). For women in households with no car, shopping and escort journeys are typically made on foot. In families with one car, walking is still the main mode of transport during the day, with the car only taking over during the evening (see Table 9.5).

Table 9.5: Housewives' Day-Time Transport Patterns, Great Britain, 1975

% use between 9.0a.m. & 5.0p.m.	Households with no car	Households with one car	Households with two or more cars
Car	8	37	68
Bus	16	6	2
Walk	73	55	27
Other	3	2	3
	100	100	100

Source: Department of Transport (1979) *National Travel Survey: 1975/6 Data*, published in Pickup, L. (1981) *Housewives' Mobility and Travel Patterns*, p.12.

Housewives form a significant proportion of bus travellers and in all age groups women are heavier users of buses than men (Potter, 1982: 8). Between 9 a.m. and 5 p.m., about one third of bus users are housewives (Pickup, 1981:13). Bus use among women, however, varies with the age of their children. A study of mobility in suburban areas found that mothers with children under three used the bus on average only once a week, while mothers with children between three and five travelled by bus twice a week (Hillman, Henderson and Whalley, 1974).

Although women with children rely on walking and on public transport to meet their commitments outside the home, both are associated with problems. In Hillman, Henderson and Whalley's study, women travelling on foot with their children found problems with carrying shopping and manoeuvring prams in congested streets and across busy roads. The study uncovered greater problems among bus users. Most frequently mentioned was the unreliability of the service and the high cost of bus fares (ibid.). As other surveys have noted, the cost of public transport has risen significantly faster than the Retail Price Index over the last decade (Potter, 1982). Such rises present particular problems to users on low and fixed incomes, like housewives and pensioners, who depend heavily on public transport. Significantly, in the context of the problems that travelling on foot and by bus present to mothers with children, the study by Hillman, Henderson and Whalley noted that mothers experienced few problems travelling with young children by car.

The evidence on travel patterns among women, in employment and with children, bears directly on their health care roles. As we have seen, how public transport is organised (its availability, its cost, its design) increases or reduces women's opportunities to secure employment and to reach the services which professionals regard as so important for family health. How private transport is distributed, between and particularly within families, similarly acts to help or hinder women's efforts to promote health. Transport policies, it appears, must be incorporated within the framework of a policy for family health.

9.5 TRANSPORT AND HEALTH

While 'income and health', 'housing and health' and 'food and health' are familiar couplings, the role of transport in shaping family health has not been systematically explored. However, the necessary research is available to launch such an exploration.

It is known, for example, that public transport provides a safer means of travel for passengers and pedestrians than private cars (Smith, 1981). Per mile travelled, ten times more occupants (drivers and passengers) die in private cars than in buses and coaches; five times more die in private cars than on British Rail and the London underground. The pattern holds true for pedestrians: per mile travelled, two and a half times more pedestrians are killed or seriously injured by private cars than by buses and coaches (ibid.).

Safety is not the only consideration for parents working for family health. Cost, convenience and the problems of travelling with young children are also major concerns. Many of the journeys women make are to secure resources for health: they are journeys to buy groceries, journeys to play-groups and journeys to the doctor. Many of these journeys, too, are made with, and on behalf of, children. Private transport, while more dangerous, offers distinct advantages to mothers. However, although the majority of Britain's households have a car, few women have access to the family car for their health journeys. Health-travel is concentrated during the hours of nine to five, when women are effectively car-less. Public transport, where available, is not always an acceptable alternative. The cost of public transport, and the problems it presents for travellers with children, lead many women to prefer to walk. As a result, women with children, like pensioners, become heavily reliant on local facilities. Moreover, 'local' takes on a precise geographical meaning. Local facilities, community services and neighbourhood amenities are those within walking distance with children under three. As Pickup notes, low mobility among mothers need not mean that their access to resources is restricted, if good facilities are available in the locality (Pickup, 1981:14). However, the tendency to concentrate food retailing outlets and medical services in fewer, larger centres serves to distance the carers from the resources they need to fulfil their responsibilities.

This centralisation of family services means that the delivery of care to families increasingly occurs in a symbolic sense only: parents must travel and collect the supplies of food and medical care that they need for their families. In such circumstances, the costs and benefits of securing these supplies are often finely balanced. For poor families in particular, a rational decision may be one which rejects professional care. The mother may choose instead to invest her limited reserves of time, money and energy in other areas of family health: in protecting the family diet, for example, or in her keeping her children warm.

How carers see and weigh up their responsibilities, and how they attempt to meet them within the often-restricted confines of the home, is the subject of Chapters 10 and 11.

Part IV
RESPONSIBILITIES FOR FAMILY HEALTH

10 Caring in Sickness and Health

10.1 INTRODUCTION

The question of what families do to promote and protect their health has been the major theme of this book. Earlier chapters have addressed various aspects of family responsibility, describing the patterns of health and the context of family health care. They have examined how the social environment impinges on family life, influencing the way in which the responsibilities of income-production and home maintenance are allocated between the sexes. They have described, too, how the economic facts of family life determine the distribution of such health resources as fuel, food and transport between and within families.

In their concern with the context of family health, these early chapters only obliquely describe the content of health care in the home. It is this question of content that is considered in Chapters 10 and 11. These chapters describe the reality of caring as an everyday routine which, literally and metaphorically, keeps the family going.

In sharpening our focus on the domestic domain, it is all too easy to dispense with the social environment and see health as a product of family life. There is a marked tendency in much of the literature to adopt this narrower, and more myopic, perspective. The major reviews of the family's role in health and health care by Litman (1974) and Schwenk and Hughes (1983) are pitched at the level of culture rather than material reality. While reference is made to sex roles within the home and to the economic forces beyond it, the family is seen as a unit which can be analysed separately from either.

In order to provide a perspective on health care which takes account of both culture and social structure, Chapters 10 and 11 are concerned with everyday areas of health responsibility. The section below outlines these daily activities, with the main sections of the two chapters examining them in more detail.

10.2   RESPONSIBILITIES FOR HEALTH: A TYPOLOGY

When we look at family life, it is sometimes difficult to see that a large part of what parents do is work for health. We tend to describe family activities in ways which obscure their health-promoting (or health-threatening) dimensions. For example, we use the term 'socialisation' in our accounts of childrearing, yet it is a term which fails to convey the fact that parents ensure the survival as well as the socialisation of their children. As a result, we can emphasise the importance of mothers in shaping the minds of children, while remaining blind to their role in building and repairing their bodies. In a similar way, we can describe the nature of housework, but not record how much of the housewife's labours are devoted to maintaining the family's health rather than maintaining their home. It is the shopping, the cooking, the laundry and the 'being with' activities which consume most in terms of time, money and energy (Thomas and Shannon, 1982:16). By comparison, cleaning the home is an activity which occupies a comparatively small part of the carer's workload, particularly for mothers with young children.

To refocus our vision on the myriad health-tasks that families accomplish every day, it is useful to identify some of them formally. Chapters 10 and 11 examine five areas of activity: providing for health, nursing the sick, teaching about health and illness, mediating professional help and coping with crisis. As outsiders looking into the family, we can see these tasks as separate; experiencing them as insiders, they are likely to merge indistinguishably, becoming part of what we know and take for granted as normal family life.

Providing for health involves all the basic domestic activities we associate with the maintenance of a home. It involves the provision of a materially-secure environment: warm, clean accommodation where both young and old can be protected against danger and disease. It involves the purchase of food and the provision of a diet sufficient in quantity and quality to meet their nutritional needs. Providing for health involves, too, the provision of a social environment conducive to normal health and development. It means, for example, orchestrating social relations within the home to minimise the health-damaging insecurities that can arise when these relations go awry.

Nursing the sick places on the carer the additional domestic responsibilities created by illness in the family. Much of the work of caring for a relative during a period of illness is similar to that demanded during health: meals must be cooked, beds made, laundry washed and shopping done. However, there is likely to be more of it. Nursing the sick is a more constant and labour-intensive responsibility than caring for the well. It is also a responsibility which demands closer and more frequent contact with outsiders, and with health professionals in particular. These differences typically involve an added financial burden. The costs of heating, food, laundry and transport are all likely to be higher during periods of family sickness.

Teaching about health is a responsibility which is accomplished, intentionally or unintentionally, as part of the carer's day. In providing for family health or in treating family illness, parents are inevitably working as health educators. In setting standards of diet and hygiene, for instance, parents are not only facilitating health in a biological sense: they are transmitting a culture in which health and illness can be understood. Looking after yourself and looking after children involves teaching by example.

Caring for the family is not an exclusively home-based activity. Health responsibilities include *mediating with outsiders*. In particular, they involve contact with professional welfare workers: the doctor and health visitor, the social worker and the district nurse, the school nurse and the health education officer.

In identifying four areas of health responsibility, artificial boundaries are imposed on what, in practice, are inseparable activities. As observers of family life, we can abstract health education from health care, we can distinguish nursing the sick from seeing the doctor. Living within the family, the four are subsumed within a domestic routine which manages, most of the time, to integrate care, treatment, education and professional support.

Integrating responsibilities is not always a straightforward matter. While responsibilities can be listed on a page, in real life they do not always dovetail so neatly. Instead, as earlier chapters have reported, responsibilities are often in conflict. In meeting the children's need for food, the diet of the parents can suffer: in providing a car for the male breadwinner, the children's access to medical services is restricted. Caring is thus about reconciling as well as meeting commitments; it is about containing demands and conserving supplies to ensure that needs and ends meet. Coping with conflict and *coping with crisis* thus constitutes a fifth, and perhaps most vital, area of activity for the family carers.

Taking care of the family brings with it a distinctive life-style for mothers and others who assume the responsibilities of the housewife. This life-style is described in the sections which follow. Caring, however, is more than a style of life; it is a labour of love (Graham, 1983: b). Emotions, as well as activities, lie at the heart of caring relationships. To commit yourself to care for your family is thus a statement of who you are, as well as what you do. Caring — as a married mother, lone father, dutiful daughter — is not only your occupation; it is a part, and often the central part, of your identity.

Because caring is an expression of intimacy, tenderness and loyalty, the rewards of caring can be great. But because carers do indeed care, there are less positive consequences too. A mother's love and sense of commitment can provoke anxiety that things may go wrong and guilt and self-recrimination when they do. Responsibility is felt in an acute and highly personal way. It is this feeling of responsibility that emerges as a recurrent motif in surveys of carers and in the accounts that carers give of their experiences (Graham, 1982: a). Parents, and mothers especially, identify themselves as the person 'who is answerable for whatever happens' (Hughes et al., 1980: 26).

It is with this sensitivity to the position and perspective of carers that Chapters 10 and 11 should be read.

Over and above the physical demands and restrictions that mothers face, there is the added burden for most of feeling continually and ultimately responsible for the health, development and happiness of their children. However much help a mother may get in bringing up her children, she is still likely to feel that she is the person beyond whom there is no resource or appeal and who is answerable for whatever happens.[1]

10.3 PROVIDING FOR HEALTH

The most fundamental responsibility carried by mothers is that of providing for health. It is the most life-sustaining and labour-intensive aspect of women's health work; the activity through which the basic material resources of housing, fuel, food and transport are used to make healthy children and healthy parents. Providing for health keeps the family going. Moreover, it provides the setting in which the other health responsibilities are pursued: nursing the sick, teaching for health and mediating with professionals.

Yet, strangely, the maintenance of family health is the least well-documented area of lay health care. Despite the popular and political interest in the family, we know very little about the physical and psychological labour of sustaining human life. While the family is recognised to be Britain's primary and most important health care institution, we remain surprisingly ignorant about how it works.

What we do know is drawn from studies which have focussed on components of women's health role. Some of these studies have separated out the tasks of housework, childrearing, food preparation and the care of the sick and handicapped, surveying each on its own (Oakley, 1974; Newsom and Newsom, 1970; Murcott, 1982:a). Meanwhile, other surveys have concerned themselves with the psychological attributes of caring, surveying women's knowledge of and attitudes to various dimensions of health-maintenance. Research has described women's attitudes to health and the control of illness, to childrearing and to the professional services which assist parents in their health and childcare responsibilities (McKinlay, 1973; Pill and Stott, 1982; Blaxter and Paterson, 1982). While the studies are illuminating, they describe only fragments of caring. In reality, health attitudes are embedded in domestic activities, and these activities — shopping, cooking, washing, watching, waiting — are moulded by the practical constraints of time, space and money.

Describing what health provision and health maintenance involve is difficult not only because they lack clear boundaries. Carers find it hard to describe their day also because it remains largely unseen. Maintaining health is most in evidence when it is not done: when clothes and faces are left unwashed, rooms and hair are untidy, and children are ill-disciplined and noisy. When the mother works successfully to maintain the standards of dress, decor and decorum, her labour is at its most invisible (Graham, 1982: b).

I do not change things. The work I do changes nothing; what I cook disappears, what I clean one day must be cleaned the next.[2]

Although well-hidden, it is nonetheless possible to identify the contours of this elusive activity. Two features, in particular, stand out. Firstly, providing for health imposes a distinctive time-structure on carers. Secondly, it is an activity which involves routines which are both constant and constantly changing.

Firstly, studies give us a sense of the time and pace of health-work. Surveys conducted over the course of this century suggest that full-time housewives spend well over fifty hours a week on housework and childcare (Oakley, 1974:94).

Time budgets show that the total time women spend on their domestic tasks has declined very little in the last half-century ... What has changed is the way in which their time is distributed between the various tasks: the proportion of time spent on childcare has increased and the time spent on cooking and cleaning has decreased. Standards change over time and broadly speaking change upwards.[3]

Contained within the working week of housewives are long working days. In one study of activity patterns in a working-class housing estate, the working day of employed men spanned nine hours (of which less than one hour was domestic chores). The working day of women was typically between twelve and fifteen hours long (Cullen and Phelps, 1975:52). Women in employment devoted less time to housework, but had a longer working day than women who were full-time housewives.

Cullen and Phelps found that it was not only the hours of work that distinguished the men and women in their sample. The distribution of work-effort through the day was also characteristically different for the two sexes. They found that the husband's work-activities were concentrated between 7.00 a.m. and 6.00 p.m., peaking at 10.00 a.m. and 3.00 p.m. The work-patterns of their wives were more complex. Like their husbands, the housewives rose early and were busiest during the morning. As other surveys suggest, mornings are the time for housework and laundry, they are also times for shopping and escort journeys (Oakley, 1974: 100-12). In Cullen and Phelps' study, the domestic peak fell gradually in the afternoon, but rose sharply again in the late afternoon and early evening. By 7.30 p.m., one third of the housewives, and one third of the women in employment, were still working in the home.

One thing I've learned is that there is a lot more to being a housewife than I thought . . . I didn't know it before, and now I look at the house in a completely different way. I used to sit down and relax, now I sit down and think, oh that needs doing or that needs dusting. It's an enormous job, it's a twenty-four-hour job.[4]

This pattern of activity is dictated by the needs of the family and by a system of public provision of services which assumes that clients and customers are available during normal working hours. It is in the morning and early evening that many of the carers' responsibilities are clustered. In the early hours of the day, cooking, eating, dressing and escorting to school must all be accomplished before 9.00 a.m. Similarly, in the space of a few hours in the early evening, cooking, eating, washing up, bath-times and bed-times have all to be completed. The early evening, too, is the time when the family car is most likely to be available. Shopping and fetching are thus often added to the list of activities for this heavily-booked period of the day.

Given this task overload, it is perhaps not surprising to find the early evening identified as the crisis-time by carers. It is at this time, when the mother has been working for upward of ten hours, that children and husbands are tired and hungry also. Significantly, it is in the early evening that casualty departments receive most of their child casualties. The peak time for a child to attend an accident and emergency department is between 7.00 and 8.00 p.m. (Royal College of General Practitioners, 1982: 4).

The conflicting pressures build up through the day and often come to a head in the early evening when the husband returns home from work: 'I like to have David's tea on and ready when he comes home. And very often, that is when the baby's at his worst. And David comes home to no tea and these two screaming their heads off and me going up the wall'.[5]

After the pressurised period between 4.00 p.m. and 8.00 p.m., there is the relative calm of late evening. For many, this brief period of relaxation is essential for their physical and emotional regeneration.

My older boy has to go to bed at ten o'clock. I've been coping with things all day long and I want that hour for myself ... I say to him he has to go to bed. 'What are you going to do, Mum?'
'I'm not going to do a goddamned thing. I'm going to sit here ... I want to sit here by myself.'[6]

Like time alone, sleep is also seen as essential for calm and competent caring. Yet sleep too is a scarce resource. With young children and disabled relatives, disturbed nights are typical (Graham and McKee, 1980; Nissel and Bonnerjea, 1983). In the study of early motherhood that I conducted with Lorna McKee, nine in ten mothers were chronically tired at one month after the birth of their baby, and tiredness, along with the baby crying, were the two recurrent motifs in mother's accounts of their feelings of anger and exhaustion.

[Two mothers with 6 week old babies.]
'I shouted at him t'other night, he was getting all upset. I'm more tired than anything. If I could get a bit more sleep I don't think I'd be so irritable.'
  'I was really tired — normally I can wake, feed him and go back — but this night I just couldn't wake up. And he was crying and I'd fed him and he still wasn't settling — this was when I was breast feeding and he wasn't getting enough ... (She goes downstairs and makes a bottle while he continues to scream) I changed him and fed him the bottle and he still wouldn't go back. And I went to get another nappy cos he'd wet again. And I just went and sat down with my head in the airing cupboard and I just started to cry "Oh for God's sake, shut up!" That was just that night. It was just being tired. If I can get my sleep, I can cope with it.'[7]

Health care does not only impose a particular time-structure on the carer. Her day is distinctive in a second respect. Caring is simultaneously both a highly routinised and a constantly changing activity. Each day the mother is likely to perform the same operations for the same people. Yet every day her family has changing needs, demanding new responses.

The activity of housework, the cleaning and tidying and cooking, is interwoven with the work which relates directly to human beings. Housework can never be a normal job routine because emotion erupts in its midst. Crisis and turmoil mean that the woman has to drop everything and put Humpty together again.[8]

A commitment to order and routine, and an acceptance of change and chaos, are integral elements in the psychology of caring. It is the latter aspect, the capacity to perceive and adapt to changing needs, which has been highlighted in research on caring. Sensitivity to the needs of others has been identified as particularly important in the parent-child relationship (Baker Miller, 1976; Chodorow, 1978).

People who are most attuned to psychological growth are those most closely in touch with it, those who are literally forced to keep changing if they are to continue to respond to the altering demands of those under their care. For an infant and then a child to grow there must be someone who can respond to the child. As the child grows, one's responses must change accordingly. What sufficed today will not suffice tomorrow. The child has come to a different place, and the caretaker must move to another place too. If you are the caretaker you keep trying to do so. Thus, in a very immediate and day-to-day way women *live* change.[9]

10.4 NURSING THE SICK

Those responsible for caring for the family in health are also the ones responsible for care during sickness. Carpenter, in an American study, found that it was mothers and not fathers who typically provided home nursing for sick children (Carpenter, 1980: 1210). Among parents in employment, women reported three times as many hours of work lost as men because of family illness, and these absences were due primarily to children's illness (ibid.). As another survey of women's informal nursing concluded, a mother's care 'is personal and in the right place at the right time' (Auster, Leveson and Sarachek, 1966: 411).

Women's role during family illness extends from the initial perception of symptoms to the provision of long-term care for the sick and the disabled. Although sensitivity to others has been identified by psychologists, it is only recently that the diagnostic and adaptive skills of parents have been recognised within medicine. Spencer's careful study of parental responses to childhood illness has described the way in which mothers quickly notice changes in their babies' appearance and behaviour. The appearance of a 'look' in the baby's eyes is particularly important in this initial diagnosis. When confronted with these signs parents decide whether or not their child is ill, constantly reviewing their diagnosis over time, as the patterns of symptoms change. (Spencer, 1980, and forthcoming).

Parents used skills that have gained scant recognition among health professionals and that do not appear to depend on detailed knowledge of medically-accepted signs and symptoms of illness ... These skills appear to be the basis of the vital process of recognition and assessment by parents of illness in their infants.[10]

Diagnostic skill is also in evidence when the symptoms are those of disability, rather than illness. A series of studies have suggested that parents suspect handicap before medical diagnosis confirms it; in fact, parental diagnosis often triggers the decision to seek professional advice. In a study of children with Down's Syndrome, nearly two thirds of the mothers suspected their child was disabled and sought confirmation rather than diagnosis from their doctor (Cunningham and Sloper, 1977). Similarly, in a more recent study of mothers caring for severely disabled children at home, it was typically the mother who first recognised the handicap. In six out of ten cases, initial diagnosis was by the mother: in three out of ten cases, by the hospital doctor (Ayer, 1982). In the remainder, it was the midwife, family doctor and/or the school who first recognised the handicap.

The possibility of handicap is an anxiety that haunts many parents. In pregnancy, particularly, mothers are likely to be anxious in case their baby will not be 'all right'. In our study of pregnancy and motherhood, nine in ten mothers reported that they worried about their babies' normality (Graham and McKee, 1980). For many women, their worries had a specific focus: on disabilities that they may have inadvertently caused themselves. It was not simply the possibility of having a handicapped baby that concerned them, but the possibility of finding that they were responsible for the disability (Graham, 1977). Blaxter and Paterson, in their study of Scottish mothers, noted a similar anxiety: 'rather than guilt, it was *responsibility* which they felt so heavily' (Blaxter and Paterson, 1982: 86, their italics).

I suppose I felt if he was going to be abnormal and there was nothing I could do about it, that was that. But if it was going to be abnormal through my neglect, then that was inexcusable.[11]

When a baby is born with disabilities, care again falls largely on the mother (Wilkin, 1979). Disability almost invariably increases the burden of care and extends the duration of caring. Because disabled children are less independent, they continue to need help with washing, dressing, feeding and toileting long after other children have mastered these skills. As Baldwin and Glendinning note in their study of severely disabled children, 'severe disablement in a child typically prolongs the duration of dependencies, normal in infancy and early childhood, long beyond their appropriate chronological ages. Developmental "milestones" may be delayed, or never attained at all' (Baldwin and Glendinning, 1983: 55). In addition, Baldwin and Glendinning found that disabled children are often in poor health and vulnerable to illness.

While a mother is quick to identify and respond to symptoms of illness and disability in others, she appears less assiduous in monitoring her own health. Her role in caring for others appears to blunt her sensitivity to her own needs. Being ill makes it difficult for individuals to maintain their normal roles and responsibilities: since the mother's roles and responsibilities are particularly indispensable, mothers are reluctant to be ill. In Campbell's study of mother-child pairs, for example, mothers were much more likely to identify conditions listed by the researcher as indicating illness in their children than in themselves (Campbell, 1975: b: 119). They were also much more inclined to get in contact with the doctor when their children were unwell. A study of working-class mothers in south Wales similarly found that carers clearly recognised the constraints on them adopting the sick role (Pill and Stott, 1982). 'A common theme was "of course, I hardly ever go to the doctor" or "I only go for myself when it is absolutely necessary" contrasted with "I always take the children straight away if I'm a bit worried" (ibid., 1982: 49). It is possible that women overestimate the extent to which they are the lynchpins of the family. However, researchers have found that when mothers are (or allow themselves to be) sick, the quality of care in the family suffers (Litman, 1974: 506).

I think with a family you can't afford to be ill, you know what I mean? You think, well you'll be ill after you've cooked the tea. But, of course, if you're very ill, you'd have to give up — but I never have.[12]

I wish I knew what you mean by being sick. Sometimes I felt so bad I could curl up and die but I had to go on because of the kids who have to be taken care of and besides, we didn't have the money to spend for the doctor. How could I be sick? Some people can be sick anytime with anything, but most of us can't be sick, even when we need to be.[13]

Illness in the carer presents particular problems for one parent families. With the parent ill, the responsibility of both income-production and childcare are left unmet. Marsden, in his study of single mothers, noted how mothers were deterred from seeking medical help for their health problems because there was no one to take over. Similarly, in Evason's more recent study of lone parents, fear of becoming ill was one of the recurrent worries mentioned by her respondents. When asked what was the problem uppermost in their minds, one mother replied, 'I'm much better off now but if anything happened to me what would become of the kids? That's my biggest problem. While I'm healthy and here I could always manage, but if I was unfortunate enough to lose my health I don't know how I would cope'. Another replied simply 'Dying — I worry in case anything happens to me — what would happen to the children?' (Evason, 1980: a: 81-3).

There's something inside [me] that needs doing. And some nights I'll have the most awful pains when I turn over in bed. But you see I had a little talk with the children and said perhaps they could go into a Home while I went in the Infirmary, but they started crying, so I have not mentioned it again.[14]

Mothers play a prominent part in defining and coping with illness. They also play a pivotal role in the decision to seek medical care. Their mediating role, discussed in outline in this section, is described in more detail in the next chapter.

NOTES

1. Hughes, M. et al. (1980) *Nurseries Now*, p.26.
2. Tax, M. (1970) *Woman and Her Mind*, p.7.
3. Land, H. (1981) *Parity begins at home*, pp.16-17.
4. A lone father in Itzin, C. (1980) *Splitting Up*, p. 41.
5. Graham, H. (1980: a) 'Family influences in early years on the eating habits of children' in Turner, M. (ed.) *Nutrition and Lifestyles*, p.173.
6. Weiss, R. (1979) *Going It Alone*, Ch.3.
7. Graham, H. (1980: b) 'Mothers' accounts of anger and aggression towards their babies' in Frude, N. (ed.) *Psychological Approaches to Child Abuse*, p.45.
8. Rowbotham, S. (1973) *Woman's Consciousness, Man's World*, p.73.
9. Baker Miller, J. (1976) *Towards a New Psychology of Women*, p.58.
10. Spencer, N. (1979) 'An education for health educators?' in Anderson, D., Perkins, E. and Spencer, N. *Who Knows Best in Health Education?* Leverhulme Health Education Project, p.21.
11. Graham, H. (1982: a) 'Perceptions of Parenthood', *Health Education Journal*, Vol. 41.4: 119.

12. Pill, R. & Stott, N. (1982) 'Concepts of illness causation and responsibility: some preliminary data from a sample of working class mothers', *Social Science and Medicine*, Vol.16: 50.
13. Koos, E. (1954) *The Health of Regionville: What the People Felt and Did About It*, p.30.
14. Marsden, D. (1973) *Mothers Alone*, p.145.

11 Teaching about Health, Seeking Help and Coping with Crisis

11.1 INTRODUCTION

Taking responsibility for the family's well-being involves more than the provision of a secure home environment and the care of the sick. Health work covers both health education and professional liaison as well. In the social scientists' code, the mother is the primary agent in health socialisation; she is also the motivating force behind lay referral and medical utilisation. Sections 11.2 and 11.3 discuss these two aspects of the carer's role.

Section 11.4 describes the fifth and most enduring aspect of caring identified in Chapter 10: dealing with crisis. Domestic management involves not only specific health responsibilities; it involves, too, being responsible for ensuring that these responsibilities are met. Being-responsible-for-responsibilities requires an ability to deal quickly and effectively with conflicts, shortages and emergencies. In the language of everyday life, it means being able to cope.

11.2 TEACHING ABOUT HEALTH

Health education is unlikely to be a formal part of the carer's day. Instead, it is an ubiquitous aspect of the care that mothers provide for their husbands and children. In cooking, mothers demonstrate many subtle messages about the value of food and family life. In the organisation of bed-times, mothers convey to their children ideas about their body and its need for sleep, and ideas, too, about her needs for rest and for privacy once the day's work is done.

While health education is likely to be ingrained into the domestic routines of health provision, it is possible to separate the two analytically. The question of how illness concepts and health orientations develop is an important one for policies concerned with changing individual attitudes and practices. But surprisingly, the family's health experiences and their effect on the child have received little attention (Mechanic, 1964: 445: Campbell, 1975: a: 93; Blaxter, 1981: 181). However, the few studies which have been conducted address a basic assumption of health education: that children acquire health beliefs from and in the family, through the process of primary socialisation. In particular, the studies question whether health learning is a process controlled by the mother.

A study of mother-child pairs in the 1960s found that children's attitudes to health and illness could not be explained in terms of the attitudes of their mothers (Mechanic, 1964: 447). A more carefully-controlled study by Campbell comes to similar conclusions (Campbell, 1975: a and b; 1978). In a sample of 260 children and their mothers, Campbell found that a mother's health beliefs were a poor predictor of those of her child. He concludes that the data 'do not support the view that children's definitions of illness directly result from maternal tuition. A more casual learning process may be involved, one in which mother's perspectives may make a difference only insofar as they impinge on and thus modify children's relevant experiences' (ibid, 1975: a: 99). However, while ruling out the possibility that children learn their health concepts directly from their mothers, Campbell notes that children's attitudes do vary according to the social background of the family. He concludes that children's perspectives are shaped, not directly through parental instruction, but indirectly through the common experiences that a shared position in the class structure brings.

This conclusion is endorsed by the recent SSRC/DHSS research on deprivation and disadvantage. In *Mothers and Daughters*, Blaxter and Paterson (1982) studied a group of mothers and their married daughters who were themselves mothers. Their data suggest that attitudes are not transmitted in any simple way from generation to generation. Instead, Blaxter and Paterson found that similar attitudes existed only when, and to the extent that, the mothers and daughters shared experiences born of a common environment.

These three studies, by Mechanic, Campbell and Blaxter and Paterson, suggest that while mothers (like the rest of us) transmit health messages, their children do not necessarily absorb them. Instead, the learning process is mediated not through the family's health culture, but more directly through experience. A child's experience of health, in turn, is shaped by the material environment in which the child lives, a material environment, as we saw in Chapter 3, represented in the social class position of the head of household. For families in poverty, everyday experiences are commonly ones of physical deprivation and mental stress.

The children, in the process of growing up, have many shared experiences. They live in overcrowded conditions, being members of large families; their homes are inadequate by current standards; the neighbourhoods are rough and disliked by most of those who have to live in them. They experience poverty ... and they lack experiences encountered as normal by others around them. Most, if not all, the children have first-hand knowledge of illness, disability, accidents and mental stress expressed in a variety of symptoms. They must learn, in growing, to come to terms with or contain the situations of stress to which they are subjected day by day ... Events in these children's lives repeat themselves and form a pattern and thus become part of what appears to them to be the hazardous business of living ... The draining of human energy and potential is the element that outweighs all others and has an overpowering effect on the growth of children that no other element can counter-balance.[1]

11.3 MEDIATING PROFESSIONAL HELP

Taking responsibility for family health commits the carer to activities beyond as well as within the home. As the principal carer, the mother acts not only as the home nurse, home doctor and home tutor. She is also the person in contact with the professionals who perform these roles in the public domain. Typically it is mother who seeks out health professionals; she is the one, too, who is sought out by them.

Normally, and by preference, the state deals not with individuals but with *families*. More often than not it deals with the *woman* of the family. Who answers the door when the social worker calls? Who talks to the head teacher about the truant child? Who runs down to the rent office? The woman, wife and mother.[2]

As noted in Chapter 9, medical consultation increasingly takes place outside the home. Even in the traditionally home-oriented services, there has been a marked shift away from domiciliary care. Health visitors, for example, are now seeing fewer children in their homes: 77% of children received domiciliary visits from health visitors in 1976 compared with 87% ten years earlier (Central Policy Review Staff, 1980: 31). Since the mid-1960s, there has been a similarly pronounced fall in the proportion of G.P. consultations taking place in the patient's home. Data from the General Household Survey suggest that the overwhelming majority of children and adults travel to their doctor when they need medical attention (Table 11.1). Given the increasing reliance on appointments made in surgery hours, the findings of the Acheson Report on *Primary Health Care in Inner London* make disturbing reading. The Acheson Report found that nearly half (43%) of Inner London practices were not directly contactable even during normal working hours (Acheson, 1981).

Table 11.1: Doctor Consultations: By Site of Consultation: Great Britain, 1980 (Number in sample = 4188)

Persons who consulted a GP (NHS) in the 14 days before interview

| Site of consultation | Age | | | |
	0-4	5-15	16-44	All ages
Surgery	75	81	92	83
Home	18	13	6	14
Telephone	13	12	6	8

Source: OPCS (1982) *General Household Survey 1980*, Table 7.14, p. 140.

When contact is established, the transactions between the informal carers and the professional health workers take two main forms. Firstly, mothers and professionals meet to ensure that preventative services reach the family, with immunisation, dental care and attendance at child health clinics being the best-researched examples. Secondly, mothers negotiate with professionals during times of illness. These meetings typically occur at the point where the resources of informal caring have been exhausted. This is where, in Zola's terms, 'the accommodation of symptoms' breaks down (Zola, 1973). In the words of the carers, it is the point where they can cope no longer. In turning to outsiders, carers are not necessarily searching for a cure. They may be searching instead for a way of alleviating suffering, in both the patient and the family. Alleviation, as we saw in our review of health resources (Chapters 6 to 9) is fundamental to women's work in the home. As the home-maker and caretaker, mothers work to relieve the stress of conditions, social and clinical, which they can neither prevent nor cure. However, while alleviation and rehabilitation are important for lay health care, they are relatively neglected areas in the medical curriculum. They are eclipsed, too, in health education, by its traditional concern with prevention and early detection (Tuckett, 1979: 55).

The decision to seek professional help, whether preventative, curative or ameliorative, is rarely taken alone. The decision-making process is one that involves other people: husbands, relatives and friends. This wider group has been identified as a 'lay referral network', a network which influences when and how to see the doctor (Friedson, 1961). Although emphasis has been placed on referral, the lay network is more accurately seen as one of carers rather than advisers (Graham, forthcoming). As we noted in the previous section, these lay caring networks are organised primarily by relatives and by female kin in particular (Abrams, 1977). Friends are more likely to act in an advisory capacity, and to advise that medical help is sought (Calnan, 1983).

The decision to seek professional help is related to the capacity of the caring network to support the sick and contain their sickness. It is a decision which, implicitly or explicitly, raises questions about the commitment and competence of the carers. These moral dimensions of illness have been identified in a wide range of studies. The picture they present, however, is a complex one. With some illnesses and with some patients, a parent's status as a carer is enhanced by securing medical help. In preventative care, particularly when it relates to children, responsible parents are identified as those who use the services. Responsible parents attend ante-natal clinics and classes, and bring their children to the dentist and the child health clinic (Graham, 1979: a). Reflecting this medical endorsement, most mothers do bring young children to the child health clinic: three quarters of the under twos in Britain are reported as attenders (Central Policy Review Staff, 1980: 31). Similarly, the majority of children are immunised against polio, tetanus, whooping cough and diptheria (Blaxter, 1981: 158).

Again, in the treatment of acute conditions in children, early attendance at the surgery and the clinic is encouraged by doctors and health visitors. Mothers, too, as we noted in section 10.4, are generally quick to refer symptoms of concern to their doctor. However, when we consider the management of chronic problems among children and the management of general health problems among adults, we find a different set of meanings attached to medical consultation. Voysey (1975), in her study of disability, found parents reluctant to involve outsiders in the process of care. Instead, they sought to organise both the labour of caring and the accounts they gave of it to outsiders in such a way that the respectability and sanctity of the family was maintained. Whatever the personal costs, the world must remain convinced that the family is coping. Similarly, Blaxter and Paterson noted in their study of *Mothers and Daughters* that women were reluctant to define their children as unhealthy, seeing it as a reflection on their mothering skills. Illness, the researchers note, is 'a moral category' (Blaxter and Paterson, 1982: 32).

Illness is equally a moral category when ascribed to the carer. Studies of motherhood have found mothers reluctant to visit their doctors about physical and emotional problems (Graham and McKee, 1980; Pill and Stott, 1982). Such evidence suggests that the rates of mental illness among women may well represent an iceberg of suffering.

If moral questions were the only ones governing the patterns of medical consultation, then we would expect preventative services to have an 100% attendance. Clearly, there are other dimensions to seeking help in which the costs and benefits of care are more finely weighed. Going to the doctor involves economic and geographical considerations as well. As we saw in Chapter 9, the spatial separation of informal and formal health care means that patients and their carers invest time and money travelling to and from medical services. Where ante-natal care is locally provided by the GP, attendance is less expensive in terms of the vital resources of time and money: where antenatal care is centralised and provided at a district hospital, the costs of attendance can be high. In my own study of pregnancy, mothers attending the hospital clinic spent twice as long travelling to and waiting at the hospital clinic as mothers receiving their antenatal care from their GP. For the first group of mothers, the trip took, on average, 123 minutes: for mothers going to the surgery, the trip took 56 minutes (Graham, 1979: b). This study, too, highlighted the problems which long journeys created for mothers travelling with children, problems noted in Chapter 9. Leaving children at home, however, is not without costs.

Attending [antenatal] classes will involve mothers with children under five in making arrangements for their care, which may be difficult, time-consuming and, in the case of a clinging toddler, emotionally exhausting. The uncertain benefits of attending classes may be outweighed by the costs in family disturbance.[3]

The costs of medical care are most apparent when a member of the family is taken into hospital. Having a child in hospital places a heavy burden on the emotional and financial resources of families. An early study, conducted in 1972, highlighted the travel costs associated with in-patient care. A survey of 1,000 children in hospital in Wales found that working-class parents visited their children less frequently than middle-class parents (Earthrowl and Stacey, 1977). The explanation did not lie in a lower commitment among working-class parents: the researchers found that parents shared almost identical beliefs about the value of visits. Instead, the difference lay in the parents' access to transport. A quarter of the working-class parents reported difficulty in obtaining transport to visit their children: and a half had difficulty paying for it.

Transport costs are only one item in the bill which families pay when their children are in hospital. A recent study of children with cancer confirmed the financial burden that in-patient care places on families in all social classes (Bodkin, Pigott and Mann, 1982). Loss of pay, plus out-of-pocket expenses (mainly travel expenses) represented an average loss of over one quarter of the family's weekly income. In the first week of treatment the financial costs were particularly high, equalling half the total weekly income for 45% of the families in the sample. Loss of the mother's earnings was the major factor contributing to the families' financial difficulties, which underlines the finding from earlier studies that it is the woman who takes the major responsibility in times of sickness.

Studies of childhood illness highlight a recurrent theme in parents' accounts of caring. The theme is one of coping with crisis: of finding ways of calmly and quietly meeting the conflicting responsibilities of parenthood.

11.4 COPING WITH CRISIS

To cope, according to the Oxford English Dictionary, means to 'contend quietly' and to 'grapple successfully'. To cope is to handle the responsibilities of everyday life with equanimity and efficiency. This idea of unobtrusive competence runs through the accounts of mothers and other carers, serving as a yardstick by which they measure their own performance.

If you've been woken half a dozen times in the night, you're just so tired and weary, you can't cope.[4]

I have a fear that I'm not going to be able to cope, because I had an easy labour last time. And there were women screaming and shouting and carrying on. I think it's the fact that perhaps I'm going to have a worse labour and show myself up. I think that's the frightening bit. That bit frightens me.[5]

Coping with caring involves more than meeting the specific health responsibilities outlined in Chapters 10 and 11. It involves reconciling them with each other and with the material constraints of family life. Coping with a family on a low income means finding ways of making ends meet and at the same time keeping the children well and contented. Coping with unemployment means exercising tighter control over the family's income without upsetting the patterns of authority which traditionally devolve from the father (McKee, 1983). Coping with the arrival of a new baby or a disabled relative involves a series of complex readjustments, in which the needs of some must be sacrificed to meet the needs of others.

Friends and family often play a crucial role in supporting parents in times of crisis. Despite the apparent drift to a nuclear family, kinship ties are still strong. In our study of 200 mothers, we found that half the mothers lived within five miles of both their own and their partners' parents. Reflecting this geographical proximity, over 60% of the mothers saw their parents or their in-laws at least once a week (Graham and McKee, 1980). A similar picture emerges in a more recent study of young families in the West Midlands. Over half the families lived in the same town as both sets of parents and nearly half met at least once a week (Bell, McKee and Priestley, 1983).

These studies indicate that kinship networks offer vital support to parents with children. However, there are limitations to the extent to which the extended family can help. Their health, their work and their home commitments, plus the costs of travel place limits on their capacity to care for others. Further, in certain circumstances, family networks appear to withdraw in the face of crisis. Parents find that friendship and contact with relatives can decline sharply after a marriage breakdown (Evason, 1980: a:52). The majority of the lone mothers in Marsden's survey 'spoke of changes in their relationship with friends and neighbours who seemed to stigmatise the family in some way, tending to isolate it' (Marsden, 1973: 111). There is evidence, too, that friends and neighbours are less willing to offer help to one parent families, particularly with childcare (Simpson, 1980). Unemployed men and their families can also find themselves isolated from former kinship ties (Marsden and Duff, 1975). Male unemployment can make it more difficult, too, for wives to keep up their former social networks (McKee, 1983). Chronic illness, like unemployment, is also associated with a weakening of the bonds which tie families to their families and relatives (EOC, 1982). In fact, studies suggest that the greater the degree of need, the smaller is the amount of external help offered (Nissel and Bonnerjea, 1983).

Coping with caring thus depends, to a considerable extent, on self-help. It depends upon a number of tried-and-tested strategies which provide the carer with a way of surviving conflicts and shortages on her own. Since most carers work in the home alone, the strategies must be ones which can be employed in the home without the assistance of outsiders. Ideally, they are measures which can enable mothers to cope with stress without leaving the room.

Several such strategies have already been discussed in earlier chapters of the book. Here, we need only to underline their significance as methods by which families, often in a very literal sense, manage to survive. Yet, many of these strategies offer a contradictory kind of support: helping and hurting the family at the same time. Although health-sustaining, coping strategies tend also to be health-threatening. By enabling the carer to cope, they appear to promote family welfare; but only by undermining individual health.

Food appears to provide such a coping strategy. In Chapter 8, we saw how sweets and treats are introduced into the daily routine to help keep the peace in situations of stress. Sweets, Kerr and Charles (1983) suggest, are used to encourage correct behaviour; instantly provided at crisis-points on buses and in the street, and held out as rewards for good behaviour in the home. Patterns of sweet-giving and sweet-eating highlight the way in which infant-feeding practices more generally are adapted to meet the exigencies of family life. This adaptation tends to involve the mother abandoning medically approved foods in favour of a diet which is considered less suitable for young babies.

The change from breast feeding to bottle feeding in the early weeks after childbirth is an example of this process. The decision to abandon breast feeding appears to reflect the problems of reconciling it with the other reponsibilities of marriage and motherhood. In our study of early motherhood (Graham and McKee, 1980), mothers often experienced a conflict of interest between their baby, their family and themselves. For example, as breast feeders they needed rest: as housewives and mothers, the other demands on their time made resting impossible. A mother with other children faced additional conflicts in her dual responsibility to her baby and her older children, with the demands of both often being at their most intense during the pressured period of early evening. Although many mothers experienced these tea-time crises, few had either the opportunity or the inclination to share the responsibility of childcare and housework with others. Instead, they had to find ways of coping with the pressures of motherhood alone. Giving up breast feeding provided one such way of coping: a way of alleviating the conflicts without disrupting the fabric of family life (Graham, 1980: a).

This time I was determined to succeed (at breast feeding). I only did it for two months with Sophie and I thought this time I am really going to persevere. But I got so tired, you can't rest when you have got two. I mean I let the housework go but I still had to do the washing and ironing and cook a meal. I just could not. I did not have enough.[6]

In the same way, a month or so later, a significant proportion of mothers decided to introduce solid foods into their babies' diet. While the majority of mothers in our study kept their babies on an all-milk diet until three months, a sizeable minority (42%) started their babies on solids earlier. For these mothers, solid foods were seen as a way of improving their babies' sleeping habits: their failure to settle after a feed, their fretfulness during the night or their tendency to wake early for feeds. Again, the key factor in the shift away from the medically-recommended feeding practices was that they placed too high a premium on the baby's health, and, in consequence, too high a cost on the mother and other members of the family. Giving the baby water when it seemed unsatisfied with its milk feed may be nutritionally preferable to thickening the feed with cereal, but it meant yet another disturbed night for the rest of the household. As one mother in our survey put it, 'the health visitor told me not to thicken his feeds but I mean they don't have to put up with his screaming' (Graham and McKee, 1980; Graham, 1980: b).

In these examples, the needs of young children are subordinated to those of older family members. However, the burden of sacrifice does not always fall on the young. With other strategies, it is the woman's health which suffers in her attempts to cope with the pressures of home and family. The role of tranquillisers in the life of the carer has already been discussed (Chapter 5). Tranquillisers, it appears, are finely tuned to the caring role, enabling the carer to remain calm in a situation where resources are few and responsibilities are many. Similarly, smoking provides a way of coping with the constant and unremitting demands of caring: a way of temporarily escaping without leaving the room.

After lunch, I'll clear away and wash up and put the telly on for Stevie (her son). I'll have a sit down on the sofa, with a cigarette and maybe a cup of tea. It's lovely, it's the one time in the day I really enjoy and I know Stevie won't disturb me.

I couldn't stop, I just couldn't. It keeps me calm. It's me one relaxation is smoking.[7]

This theme has been amplified in a recent report on women smokers, where Jacobson (1981) argues that smoking provides a means of containing (and surviving) the conflicts that spring from women's caring role. As the nature of this role becomes more complex and more anxiety-producing, women have turned to smoking 'as a safety valve, an alternative to letting off steam. They smoke not to accompany expressions of frustration and anxiety, but *instead of expressing these feelings*' (Jacobson, 1981: 32, her italics).

In doses equivalent to those obtained in smoking, nicotine can produce stimulation and arousal on the one hand and relaxation on the other. These effects depend not only on dose and individual constitution, but also on mood and situation. Thus, if we are angry or fearful its effect is to calm and sedate, but if we are bored or fatigued, it will arouse and stimulate. Nicotine serves, therefore, as a means of maintaining a constant mood in situations of stress.[8]

A central feature of the strategies examined in this section — food, tranquillisers and cigarettes — is the fact that they release, as if from nowhere, the physical and emotional energy necessary for successful coping. They provide on-the-spot relief, well-suited to the isolated position in which many carers work. The strategies provide a way of resolving, if only temporarily, two of the most stressful aspects of caring alone: conflicts of responsibility and shortage of resources. In so doing, they highlight a set of major themes about women's work within the family which have run through the previous chapters. They highlight, for example, the extent to which the organisation of family life imposes constraints on the carer, limiting her room for manoeuvre in her search for ways of promoting her family's health. The physical constraints of space and distance, the financial constraints of poverty and the limits of her own energy, force compromises in which some aspects of family health are inevitably sacrificed. In the face of inevitable compromise, what constitutes sensible and reasonable behaviour may radically change. Actions deemed irresponsible by professionals may be the only means by which mothers can act responsibly. By understanding, if only in part, the strategies by which women cope we can begin to understand how individuals and families look after themselves. We can begin to sense the responsibility of irresponsible behaviour.

NOTES

1. Wilson, H. & Herbert, G. (1978) *Parents and Children in the Inner City*, pp.103-4.
2. Cockburn, C. (1977) *The Local State*, p.58 (her italics).
3. Perkins, E. (1980) 'The pattern of women's attendance at antenatal classes: is this good enough?' *Health Education Journal*, Vol. 39, 1:8.
4. Hughes, M. et al. (1980) *Nurseries Now*, p.16.
5. Graham, H. (1982: b) 'Coping: or how mothers are seen and not heard', in Friedman, S. and Sarah, E. (eds.) *On the Problem of Men*, p.109.
6. Graham, H. (1980: a) 'Family influences in early years on the eating habits of children', in Turner, M. (ed.) *Nutrition and Lifestyles*, p.174.
7. Graham, H. (1976) 'Smoking in pregnancy: the attitudes of expectant mothers' *Social Science and Medicine*, Vol. 10: 403.
8. Royal College of Physicians of London (1977) *Smoking or Health* p.102.

Part V
CONCLUSIONS

12 Health Choices and Health Routines

12.1 INTRODUCTION

This book has drawn together the varied literature on health and health care in the home. It has done so in order to address a fundamental but neglected issue within social policy: how do parents meet their responsibilities? In confronting this issue, the book has raised, and attempted to answer, a range of questions about the organisation of family life. It has raised the question of the organisation of parental responsibilities: how do mothers and father share out the responsibilities for income production, for food preparation and housework, for childcare and for coping with illness? What are the effects of this division of labour on the lives, and the health, of parents and children? It has raised, too, the question of resources: what resources of money, time and energy do families have available for health? The book examined particularly the distribution of material resources: how are the basic necessities of money, housing, food, fuel and transport shared out among Britain's families: which families get most and which get least? How are these necessities distributed within families: is the allocation of health resources equitable and is it in line with the allocation of health responsibilities between parents?

The evidence that the book presents does not give complete answers to these questions. Nonetheless, the evidence provides sufficient information for us to gain an understanding of how parents work for family health. This understanding is essential for health and welfare professionals who are concerned that their efforts on behalf of families should support and help parents in their health work. But it has a wider political significance. The

177

social context of family care in the 1980s is a rapidly changing one. Demographic changes and changes in government policy on health and welfare are combining to increase the burden of care on families, and at the same time, reduce the burden carried by the state.

The full effects of these demographic and policy changes are yet to be registered by families and recorded by social scientists. However, it is clear that Britain's demographic structure is simultaneously increasing the number of dependents in need of care and reducing the number of potential carers able and willing to work unpaid in the community. On the one hand, more disabled children are surviving into adulthood and more elderly people are reaching and living beyond their 'three-score years and ten'. On the other, the changing patterns of marriage and women's employment have reduced the pool of potential female care-givers. While the evidence on the effects of women's employment has been accumulating since the 1960s, we have yet to witness the full impact of divorce and separation on carers and their elderly and disabled dependents. But the evidence suggest that the fragmenting of the kinship network which typically follows separation will leave women with less support. It will also leave fewer carers for the step-grandmothers and step-grand-fathers of the next generation (Walker, 1983).

Aware of the problems that they face in coping with the responsibilities of parenthood, parents are likely to become increasingly worried about their capacity to care for their relatives who are reaching the end of their life. It is a concern shared by professionals working in both the state and the voluntary sector (Oliver, 1983). Their concern does not only relate to the demographic changes in the family. It has a second focus, stemming more directly from changes in the welfare state. Current Conservative social policies are designed to enhance the caring capacity of families, to enable them to do more for themselves and for others in the community. An implicit assumption of such policies is that the family could care more than it does, and with less material support from the statutory services. While the informal sector of welfare is currently seen as an alternative to the publicly-funded structures of the welfare state, there has been little discussion of whether female relatives, friends and neighbours have the capacity to house and care for those no longer supported by the state. A range of policies designed to limit public investment in income maintenance,

?essay quote?

housing, transport, school meals and the National Health Service are being promoted, but can families do more with less? Can they take on additional responsibilities with less state support than they currently receive, and still keep together and keep healthy?

The answer from this book must be no. The weight of evidence that it presents suggests that any further reduction in the infrastructure of state support can only be at the cost of many carers and dependents. In simple terms, more care by the family is likely to mean less health for the family. Since the burden of family care falls primarily on women, more care by families is likely to have the severest consequences on women's mental and physical welfare.

This chapter highlights some of the reasons why a further shift towards family care would threaten rather than facilitate parents' efforts to protect family health. It summarises, in the section below, the evidence of the book on how families work for health. The final section considers two key concepts in the debate on health and the family, responsibility and choice, examining what these concepts mean in the context of the everyday lives of mothers and children.

12.2 HOW FAMILIES CARE

A dominant theme in recent debates about the family is that families have ceased to care for their kith and kin. The development of professional services, and publicly-funded professional services most especially, is seen to have taken over activities once performed by families. As a result, self-reliance has been eroded, leaving parents and children no longer as able or as willing to look after themselves. While some level of external support is necessary for the maintenance of the family, the balance is seen to have tipped towards undermining the family through too much rather than too little support.

The book has addressed the question of family responsibility directly. The evidence it reviews suggests that the family, as an institution for care, convalescence and rehabilitation, is not dead. Kinship networks and the immediate family in particular continue to meet a variety of health needs. Families provide for health, teach for health and absorb at least some of the additional costs — financial, physical and emotional — created by illness. However, in meeting these obligations, families draw their support from many sources, which are themselves under increasing pressure. Stress and ill-health in the home thus figure as a consequence of shortages in the support structure of family life.

What are the sources of support on which families depend for their survival? Three have been given particular prominence in the book: women's care, women's income and the external provision of goods and services. Firstly, the book records the extent to which family life, in its literal and symbolic sense, depends on the unpaid work of a parental caretaker. It depends primarily on *women's health work*. The vitality of most families rests on the fact that, despite their increasing involvement in income-production, women continue to meet the health needs of their partners and their children. While sharing the financial burden of keeping a family with their partners, women and their female relatives continue to cook, clean and care. There is little evidence to suggest a decline in the commitment of mothers to their children and their wider family: they still see themselves as 'the person beyond whom there is no recourse or appeal' (Hughes et al., 1980).

Those who care for the family tend to be responsible also for purchasing the resources necessary for caring: they buy the food, pay the rent and meet the fuel bills. Mothers thus typically act as both carer and housekeeper. They act to maintain both the health and the solvency of the household. These two roles can conflict, with the demands of caring outstripping the income available to meet them. For an increasing number of mothers, debt and ill-health present themselves as real and unavoidable alternatives, while others find themselves facing both (Burghes, 1980; Evason, 1980: a).

In some households, it is the father who is the carer and housekeeper (Hipgrave, 1982). The term used in two parent households for such arrangements is revealing. The couple 'swap roles', a phrase indicating not a sharing but a shifting of responsibilities from one parent to another. The organisation of family care typically remains the same; it is only the sex of the housekeeper which changes. The health and financial security of the family still rests on the domestic activities of a sole, and often solitary, carer. Since the art of caring involves meeting many needs simultaneously, solitary caring, whether in a one or two parent family, involves conflicts and compromises. To ensure an efficient allocation of resources, priorities have to be established: but in prioritising needs, practices are adopted which can have negative effects on health. Where demands exceed the capacity of the carer to meet them, some needs are unavoidably sacrificed for the sake of others.

A crucial determinant of the nature and scale of these health sacrifices is a second set of factors which sustain the role of the carer. As we have seen, organising health in the home demands economic as well as human resources. It demands access to an adequate and stable income. Income is necessary if parents are to provide an adequate standard of housing, food and transport for their family and if they are to be able to reach the professional services in times of need. In most households, the health-sustaining income is the income controlled by the mother: *women's income* is a vital determinant of family welfare.

While access to income is essential for informal care, a number of indicators suggest that women's incomes are often low and insecure. In particular, there are the statistics on family poverty. From these statistics, it is clear that poverty, as measured by total family income, has increased rapidly since the late 1970s. In 1979, 1.1 million families with children were living in poverty: by 1981, the figure has risen by over 50% to 1.7 million (DHSS, 1983: a). By that time, nearly one child in three in Britain was growing up on or below the poverty line. These statistics on poverty serve as a stark reminder of the number of parents who have effectively been denied the right to care adequately for their children.

Family poverty is inextricably linked to employment policy and the policies for income maintenance for those not in paid employment. Since families outside the labour market are particularly vulnerable to poverty, employment remains the most effective guarantee against both poverty and the ill-health with which it is associated. With two-person participation in the workforce increasingly becoming a condition of family life, the most direct contribution that many women can make to the welfare of the family is to go out to work. This fact, of course, turns conventional wisdom on its head. It suggests that rational, responsible, working-class mothers, may decide not to stay at home. Concerned with the most efficient and effective investment of their labour, they may seek to find and keep a paid job.

While going out to work may be the best course of action, the economic rewards can be low. As many mothers know, women workers find themselves confined to jobs where pay and conditions are poor. Women's take-home pay, even when supplemented by the earnings of a man, may not be sufficient to lift their family out of poverty. The living standards of one parent families are particularly severely affected by the low pay of women.

Where paid employment is not an option, parents and children must rely upon the state for their existence as a family with a home to live in. As Marsden (1973) observed, the living standards and health chances of families on supplementary benefit depend very directly on the minimum levels of income which governments find acceptable for the most vulnerable of its people. With a government committed to retrenchment in the welfare state, the outlook seems grim for the increasing numbers of families who are dependent on it.

But family poverty is not the only factor responsible for the low incomes of Britain's carers. It is not only a family's relation to the labour market and the welfare state which determines how much mothers can invest in family health. Research suggests that the income invested by mothers depends, secondly, on relations within the family. It depends crucially on how the money is divided up between mother and father. Compared with the data on income distribution between families, there is little empirical information on income levels within the family. We do not know in how many families the income allocated to women is insufficient to meet the bills she must pay for food, fuel, clothes, rent and transport. However, the available research suggests that poverty among women extends beyond the 1.7 million families known to be in poverty in 1981. The existence of such family poverty is likely to swell the number of families with children who are, in effect, living on incomes incompatible with health.

Tackling women's poverty must be fundamental to any strategy designed to improve the quality of the home environment. It is also fundamental to any strategy designed to bring greater equality of opportunity and life-style between men and women. Such an objective would take policy-makers beyond the boundaries of a narrowly-conceived 'health policy'. It would involve policies on employment, to increase women's opportunities to find and keep the kind of well-paid jobs available in the primary sector of the labour market. It would involve policies on social security, policies which directed increased benefits through the carer (Pond and Popay, 1983).

An adequate income is a necessary prerequisite for the maintenance of a home of sufficient quality to sustain the health of its inhabitants. However, as in other areas of life, money isn't everything. There is a third source of support on which parents depend. The data considered in this book suggest that to be self-reliant, families need a social environment which facilitates health. In particular, parents need a social environment which buttresses the care they provide for their children.

Many aspects of our social environment act to support or undermine the health work of families. Atmospheric pollution, danger from traffic, housing design and the availability of play-space all play a part. But this book has focussed on the *role of the welfare services* in family health. Attention has already been drawn in this section to the way in which the social security system provides the means of survival for an increasing number of families with children. Parents who depend for their livelihood on supplementary benefit rely heavily on the public sector for their housing. In 1981, over 60% of families on supplementary benefit were local authority tenants (Forrest and Murie, 1983: 455). In 1970, the figure was 51%. Living on state benefits is increasingly associated with living in state housing. This association has been accompanied by a deterioration in both the level of supplementary and unemployment benefit and the quality of council housing in recent years. Clearly, a greater investment in welfare benefits and in public sector housing is needed if state support is not to be increasingly linked with material deprivation and poor health.

Of course, it is not only in income maintenance and the provision of housing that the welfare state plays a vital role. The National Health Service, too, provides essential support for parents. Being universally available, the NHS is more universally used by families than the supplementary benefit system or council housing. Families with children, in particular, are heavy users of the National Health Service. It is acknowledged that the need for professional care is greatest around the time of birth, in early childhood and in old age (DHSS, 1983: b: 11). Reflecting this, health expenditure per head peaks at the beginning and end of life (ibid.). Because childhood accidents and illnesses occur both frequently and unpredictably, parents need a highly responsive network of professional services if they are to protect the health of their children. However, the evidence suggests that the professional network is not equally responsive to the needs of all families. Middle-class families receive more care and at a lower personal cost than working-class families. An appreciation of these differences has led to a search for ways of equalising access to the National Health Service. Some proposals focus on equalising the incomes of rich and poor, thus reducing the relative cost of seeking professional care among poor families (Le Grand, 1982). Other proposals concentrate on the location and delivery of the services themselves, to see if the NHS cannot be organised in such a way as to keep the costs of medical care as low as possible for families needing help. For example, attention has been drawn to the way in which parents use accident and emergency departments, ways which are not always deemed appropriate by professionals (Blaxter and Paterson, 1982: 191). The organisation of emergency care stands in contrast to the referral and appointment systems operating in other areas of the health service: access is direct and the service is quick and usually willingly given. Parents, it appears, appreciate accident and emergency departments as an alternative to the primary care available through their doctor.

Noting the importance of accessibility in the take-up of health-promoting services, this book has pointed to the role of public transport in facilitating women's work for their families. Services which are expensive to reach and expensive to use are likely to be under-utilised by parents who budget both time and money carefully. A cost-effective service, as noted in Chapter 9, has specific characteristics. It is likely to be one within walking distance of the home, or, if not close at hand, to be one served by an efficient and inexpensive system of public transport. Community health services, serving local needs, would appear to fit the criteria of a cost-effective service for parents. Shops, schools, day-care facilities and play-spaces, like health services, need to be locally-provided if they are to support the health work of mothers. Yet the tendency within both the public and private sectors is towards the increasing centralisation of supplies. Given such tendencies, the location of services and the organisation of transport become urgent matters of professional and political concern for those committed to improving family health.

In describing the role of social security, housing and public transport in family care, this book has sharpened our under-standing of the infrastructure which supports the informal health service. With such an understanding, we can begin to formulate policies which tackle the solitary nature of women's care, the poverty of the carers and the limitations of the welfare services on which they depend. We can begin, too, to assess current health policies critically. Central to these policies are the issues of responsibility and choice, issues explored in the final section of this chapter.

12.3 IRRESPONSIBILITY AND ROUTINE IN FAMILY LIFE

In encouraging families to develop health-promoting life-styles, policy-makers have emphasised the responsibilities and the choices we have in health. The concepts of responsibility and choice are particularly emphasised by the present Conservative government. By reducing the scope and scale of state support for the family, the government aims to give individuals greater control over, and choices about, their lives. The concepts of responsibility and choice play a particularly prominent part in health education, which has long been concerned with encouraging individuals to make sensible decisions about their health. What light does the material reviewed in this book shed on these important concepts?

Looking first at the question of responsibility, this book has documented the extent to which the pursuit of health tends to be a task which falls on mothers. The message of self-help and self-care is one with particular significance for women. However, in her attempt to make her family healthier, the mother must keep the costs of care within the limits of her housekeeping budget. Good health cannot be achieved at the expense of poor housekeeping, and all that it can entail for the family's longer-term security as a unit living in its own home. Disconnection of services, homelessness and the reception of children into care stand as reminders of what can happen when parents fail to reconcile caring with housekeeping. Where financial resources and domestic responsibility are evenly matched, the carer's role is considerably easier. None the less, the demands on her time and energy again make it difficult for her to establish a life-style which promotes the health of all her family.

In such circumstances, mothers tend to develop complex coping strategies. These sustain the fragile equilibrium of their everyday life, maintaining, in the words of the Royal College of Physicians of London 'a constant mood in situations of stress' (1977: 102). These coping strategies highlight a paradox of successful caring: the responsibility of irresponsible behaviour. In the professional view of family life, responsible mothers do not smoke or give their children sweets. They do not go out to work and they breast feed their babies. In the private account of family life, such behaviours may well remain the desired ones. Research suggests that mothers acknowledge the importance of breast feeding and diet in childhood (Graham, 1980: a; Kerr and Charles, 1983). However, in the context of conflicting pressures and shortage of resources, the pursuit of family welfare and the survival of the family may depend in a very real sense on routines in which individual health is jettisoned. Behaviour deemed irresponsible by outsiders becomes the means by which responsibilities can be met. For many mothers, irresponsibility is wrongly attributed: 'irresponsible' routines like smoking or sweet-giving are inescapable consequences of their commitment to family health. Complex and conflicting responsibilities can make the professionally-recommended patterns of behaviour neither rational nor responsible.

Such a paradox can only be understood in the context of family life. Turning to the concept of choice, we find again that the meaning and range of choice available to mothers is shaped by the organisation of the family. Much of the literature on health choices, however, has directed its attention away from questions of poverty and the division of labour in the home. Instead, the models explaining the health choices that people make are predominantly psychological in orientation. They locate the barriers to changing health behaviour in the belief structure of individuals. Resistance is seen as a psychological disposition: it is cognitive and affective factors which block the acquisition of new knowledge and new habits. Resistance is explained in various ways. The Health Belief Model, derived from work on patient compliance with medical advice, and the Health Locus of Control model, derived from social learning theory, have been particularly influential (Becker, Drachman and Kirscht, 1974; Rotter, 1954). In the Health Belief Model, it is the individual's perceptions of the ailment in question which is critical. In the Health Locus of Control model, the key variables are the individual's general perceptions about themselves, rather than the more specific perceptions of seriousness and risk which govern the operation of the Health Belief Model. The Health Locus of Control pinpoints as central whether or not individuals believe that they can control the outcomes of their actions. Where individuals believe they can achieve what they want (internal health locus of control), the prognosis for changes in attitude and behaviour is promising. However, where individuals believe their lives to be controlled by forces beyond their control (external health locus of control), the incentive to seek information and make changes is limited.

These models can illuminate some of the complex processes governing decision-making in the area of personal health (Tones, 1977; Pill and Stott, 1982). Both, however, are primarily concerned with attitudes and perceptions. While these dimensions are undoubtedly important, the evidence presented in this book points to the extent to which choice and change occur in a social context. Health choices are shaped by material as well as mental structures. The barriers to change are represented by the limits of time, energy and income available to parents. In such circumstances, health choices are more accurately seen as health compromises, which, repeated day after day, become the routines which keep the family going.

Understanding routines, and the constraints which bear upon them, thus appears to be essential to a broader understanding of choice and change in everyday life. Understanding routines is essential for an informed and effective health education policy: it is essential, too, for the wider debate about health and welfare. On a day-to-day level, where the struggle to establish a healthier life-style begins, the evidence suggests there is little flexibility in the routines of many families. Poverty limits a parent's command over, and thus choice about, the family's life-style. A diet high in fresh fruit may be preferred, but cannot be chosen, unless the mother reneges on equally vital health obligations: the rent and fuel bills, for example. Similarly, single parents, constrained by their childcare responsibilities as well as by their income, have little opportunity to choose the more labour-intensive methods of promoting health, like walking and jogging.

It may be conceded that choice in the context of poverty and single parenthood may have a hollow ring. But what about the majority of families, in which two parents live with their children above the poverty line? The evidence is that here, again, the space marked out for family life offers parents little opportunity for experimentation and change. Family life, as we have seen, is constrained by patterns of employment which take one parent, or more typically both parents, out of the home every day. It is constrained, too, by the system of household management, in which women are typically responsible for health purchases and health tasks. In the face of these constraints, routine can be seen to take on a distinct meaning. Routine represents the parents' attempt to maximise the restricted flexibility in their daily lives to the advantage of their family. A study of urban working-class households found that over 70% of the day (excluding sleep) was described as routine and 90% was characterised as lacking any real choice: everyday life, the study concluded, is 'a finely tuned adaptation to a relatively stable long term environment' (Cullen, 1979: 121).

From the picture of family health which emerges in this book, routine and not choice is the concept which policy-makers and professionals need to confront. For choice occurs within, and is contoured by, the routines of everyday life. These routines, it appears, mark the limit of choice available to families in different social and economic circumstances. For many families, the limits of choice are narrow and the routines, in consequence, are strict and unbending. This does not mean that individuals are implastic and resistant to change. The fact that family routines are so closely moulded to family constraints suggests, instead, that parents (and children) adapt quickly and skilfully to new situations. However, while change is possible, it involves more than will-power. The conclusion to be drawn from the evidence reviewed here is that health policies based around responsibility and choice must face the material realities in which parents work for health. Promoting genuine choice for mothers and fathers and providing effective support for their health work demands a wider political awareness of inequality and scarcity. It involves an awareness of the way in which the class structure and the structure of sexual divisions continue to shape the distribution of health resources and responsibilities. New policies to meet the health needs of families in the 1980s require the recognition that the present systems of distribution allocate fewest resources to those who have most responsibility.

Bibliography

ABRAMS, P. (1977) 'Community care: some research problems and priorities', *Policy and Politics*, 6,2: 125-51.

ACHESON, D. (1981) *Primary Health Care in Inner London*, Report of a Study Group Commissioned by the London Health Planning Consortium. (Chairman: Acheson), London: LHPC.

ADAMS, B., ASH, J. & LITTLEWOOD, J. (1969) *The Family at Home: A Study of Households in Sheffield*, London: HMSO.

ALBERMAN, E. (1977) 'Facts and Figures' in Chard, T. and Richards, M. (eds.) *Benefits and Hazards of the New Obstetrics*, London: Heinemann.

ANDERSON, D., PERKINS, E. & SPENCER, N. (1979) *Who Knows Best in Health Education?* Leverhulme Health Education Project, Occasional Paper No. 19, University of Nottingham.

ANDERSON, M. (1983: a) 'What is new about the modern family: an historical perspective' in British Society for Population Studies, *The Family*, London: OPCS.

ANDERSON, M. (1983: b) 'How much has the family changed?' *New Society*, 66, 1093: 143-6.

ARGYLE, M. (1983) 'What use are relatives?' *New Society*, 64, 1071: 293-4.

AUSTER, R., LEVESON, I. & SARACHEK, D. (1966) 'The production of health, an exploratory study', *Journal of Human Resources*, 4: 409-12.

AYER, S. (1982) *Family Care for Severely Mentally Handicapped School Children*, Unpublished Ph.D thesis, University of Hull.

BACKETT, M. (1977) 'Health Services' in Williams, F. (ed.) *Why The Poor Pay More*, London: National Consumer Council.

BAIRD, D. (1972) 'The epidemiology of low birth weight: changes in incidence in Aberdeen, 1948-1972', *Journal of Biosocial Science*, 6: 323-8.

BAKER MILLER, J. (1976) *Towards a New Psychology of Women*, Harmondsworth, Middlesex: Penguin.

BALDWIN, S. & GLENDINNING, C. (1983) 'Employment, women

and their disabled children' in Finch, J. & Groves, D. (eds.) *A Labour of Love: Women, Work and Caring*, London: Routledge & Kegan Paul.

BALLARD (1982) 'South Asian families' in Rapoport, R.N., Fogarty, M. & Rapoport, R. (eds.) *Families in Britain*, London: Routledge & Kegan Paul.

BARROW (1982) 'West Indian families: an insider's perspective' in Rapoport, R.N., Fogarty, M. & Rapoport, R. (eds.) *Families in Britain*, London: Routledge & Kegan Paul.

BAYLEY, M. (1973) *Mental Handicap and Community Care*, London: Routledge & Kegan Paul.

BECKER, M., DRACHMAN, R. & KIRSCHT, J. (1974) 'A new approach to explaining sick-role behaviour in low-income populations', *American Journal of Public Health*, 64: 205-16.

BEDALE, C. & FLETCHER, T. (1982) 'A damp site worse', *Times Health Supplement*, 12 February: 15.

BELL, C. & McKEE, L. (in progress) *Marital and Family Relations in Times of Male Unemployment* (SSRC Grant HR7939), Faculty of Management & Policy Sciences, University of Aston.

BELL, C., McKEE, L. & PRIESTLEY, K. (1983) *Fathers, Childbirth and Work*, Manchester: EOC.

BERTHOUD, R. (1981) *Fuel Debts and Hardship: A Review of the Electricity and Gas Industries' Code of Practice*, London: Policy Studies Institute.

BLAXTER, M. (1981) *Health of the Children*, London: Heinemann.

BLAXTER, M. & PATERSON, E. (1982) *Mothers and Daughters: A Three Generational Study of Health Attitudes and Behaviour*, London: Heinemann.

BODKIN, C., PIGOTT, T. & MANN, J. (1982) 'Financial burden of childhood cancer', *British Medical Journal*, 284: 1542-4.

BOWLBY, S. (1978) 'Accessibility, shopping provision and mobility' in Kirby, A, & Goodall, B. (eds.) *Resources in Planning*, London: Pergamon Press.

BOYD ORR, J. (1937) *Food, Health and Income*, London: Macmillan.

BRADSHAW, J., COOKE, K. & GODFREY, C. (1983) 'The impact of unemployment on the living standards of families', *Journal of Social Policy*, 12, 4: 433-52.

BRENNAN, M. & LANCASHIRE, R. (1978) 'Association of childhood mortality with housing status and unemployment', *Journal of Epidemiology and Community Health*, 32, 1: 28-33.

BRION, M. & TINKER, A. (1980) *Women in Housing: Access and Influence*, London: Housing Centre Trust.

BRITISH SOCIETY FOR SOCIAL RESPONSIBILITY IN SCIENCE (1979) *Asbestos Killer Dust*, London: BSSRS.

BROWN, A. (1982) 'Fathers in the labour ward: medical and lay accounts' in McKee, L. & O'Brien, M. (eds.) *The Father Figure*, London: Tavistock.

BROWN, G. & HARRIS, T. (1978) *The Social Origins of Depression*, London: Tavistock.

BROWN, M. (ed.) (1983) *The Structure of Disadvantage*, London: Heinemann.

BROWN, M. & MADGE, N. (1982) *Despite the Welfare State*, London: Heinemann.

BURGHES, L. (1980) *Living from Hand to Mouth: A Study of 65 Families Living on Supplementary Benefit*, Poverty Pamphlet 50, London: Family Service Units and Child Poverty Action Group.

BURGHES, L. (1982), 'Facts and Figures', *Poverty*, 53, December: 42-5.

BURGOYNE, J. & CLARK, D. (1983) *Making a Go of It: A Study of Step Families in Sheffield*, London: Routledge & Kegan Paul.

BURNELL, I. & WADSWORTH, J. (1981) *Children in One Parent Families*, University of Bristol: Child Health Research Unit.

BURNELL, I. & WADSWORTH, J. (1982) 'Home truths', *One Parent Times*, 8 April: 8-12.

BURR, M. & SWEETNAM, P. (1980) 'Family size and paternal unemployment in relation to myocardial infarction', *Journal of Epidemiology and Community Health*, 34: 93-5.

BUS AND COACH COUNCIL (1981) *The Future of the Bus*, London: Bus and Coach Council.

BRYNE, D., POND, C. & SULLIVAN, J. (1983) *Low Wages in Britain*, London: Low Pay Unit.

CALNAN, M. (1983) 'Social networks and patterns of help-seeking behaviour', *Social Science and Medicine*, 17: 25-8.

CALNAN, M., ABSON, E., BUTLER, J. (1982) 'In case of emergencies' *Health and Social Services Journal*, XCII, 4797: 614-17.

CAMPBELL, J. (1975: a) 'Illness is a point of view: the development of children's concept of illness', *Child Development*, 46: 92-100.

CAMPBELL, J. (1975: b) 'Attribution of illness; another double standard' *Journal of Health and Social Behaviour*, 16, 1: 114-26.

CAMPBELL, J. (1978) 'The child in the sick role: contributions of age, sex, parental status and parental values', *Journal of Health and Social Behaviour*, 19: 35-51.

CARPENTER, E. S. (1980) 'Children's health care and the changing role of women', *Medical Care*, XVIII, 12: 1208-18.

CARTWRIGHT, A. & O'BRIEN, M. (1976) 'Social class variations in health care and in the nature of general practitioner consultations' in Stacey, M. (ed.) *The Sociology of the National Health Service*, University of Keele: Sociological Review Monograph 22.

CENTRAL POLICY REVIEW STAFF AND CENTRAL STATISTICAL OFFICE (1980) *People and their Families*, London: HMSO.

CENTRAL STATISTICAL OFFICE (1981) *Social Trends 1982,* No. 12, London: HMSO.

CHAMBERLAIN, R., CHAMBERLAIN, G., HOWLETT, B. & CLAIREAUX, A. (1975) *British Births 1970, Volume 1: The First Week of Life,* London: Heinemann.

CHAMBERS, D. (1979) *Making Fathers Pay: the Enforcement of Child Support,* Chicago: University of Chicago Press.

CHODOROW, N. (1978) *The Reproduction of Mothering* ·ndon: University of California Press.

CLEAVER, J. (1981) *Fuel Costs in Households Receiving Supplementary Benefits: A Pilot Study,* South Birmingham Family Service Unit.

COCKBURN, C. (1977) *The Local State,* London: Pluto Press.

COLLEGE, M. (1981) *Unemployment and Health,* North Tyneside Community Health Council.

COLLINS, R. (1982) 'Unemployment and the division of domestic labour', Teeside Polytechnic: Department of Administrative and Social Studies.

COOPERSTOCK, R. & LENNARD, H. (1979) 'Some social meanings of tranquillizer use', *Sociology of Health and Illness,* 1, 3: 331-47.

COUNTER INFORMATION SERVICES (1981) *Women in the Eighties,* London: CIS.

COUSSINS, J. & COOTE, A. (1981) *The Family in the Firing Line: A Discussion Document on Family Policy,* Poverty Pamphlet 51, London: National Council for Civil Liberties and Child Poverty Action Group.

CULLEN, I. (1979) 'Urban social policy and the problems of family life: the use of an extended diary method to inform decision analysis' in Harris, C. (ed.) *The Sociology of the Family: New Directions for Britain,* University of Keele: Sociological Review Monograph 28.

CULLEN, I. & PHELPS, E. (1975) *Diary Techniques and the Problems of Family Life,* University College London: Joint Unit for Planning Research.

CUNNINGHAM, C. & SLOPER, P. (1977) 'Parents of Down's Syndrome babies: their early needs', *Child Care, Health and Development,* 3: 325-47.

DANIEL, W. (1980) *Maternity Rights – The Experience of Women,* London: Policy Studies Institute.

DANIEL, W. (1981) *Unemployed Flow: Stage 1: Interim Report,* London: Policy Studies Institute.

DARKE, J. & DARKE R. (1979) *Who Needs Housing?* London: Macmillan.

DAVIE, R., BUTLER, N. & GOLDSTEIN, H. (1972) *From Birth to Seven: the Second Report of the National Child Development Study (1958 Cohort),* London: Longman.

DAVIES, I. (1980) 'Perinatal and infant deaths: social and biological factors', *Population Trends*, 19, Spring: 19-21.

DEPARTMENT OF EMPLOYMENT (1982: a) *Family Expenditure Survey: Report for 1980*, London: HMSO.

DEPARTMENT OF EMPLOYMENT (1982: b) *Family Expenditure Survey: Report for 1981*, London: HMSO.

DEPARTMENT OF HEALTH & SOCIAL SECURITY (1973) *The Family in Society: Dimensions of Parenthood*, London: HMSO.

DEPARTMENT OF HEALTH & SOCIAL SECURITY (1977) *Reducing the Risk: Safer Pregnancy and Childbirth*, London: HMSO.

DEPARTMENT OF HEALTH & SOCIAL SECURITY (1978) *Eating for Health*, London: HMSO.

DEPARTMENT OF HEALTH & SOCIAL SECURITY (1981: a) *Care in Action: a Handbook of Policies and Priorities for the Health and Social Services in England*, London: HMSO.

DEPARTMENT OF HEALTH & SOCIAL SECURITY (1981: b) *Growing Older*, Cmnd 8173, London: HMSO.

DEPARTMENT OF HEALTH & SOCIAL SECURITY (1982) *Health & Personal Social Services Statistics*, London: HMSO.

DEPARTMENT OF HEALTH & SOCIAL SECURITY (1983: a) *Low Income Families, 1981:* London: DHSS.

DEPARTMENT OF HEALTH & SOCIAL SECURITY (1983: b) *Health Care and Its Costs*, London: HMSO.

DEPARTMENT OF INDUSTRY (1975) *Report on The Census of Distribution and Other Services*, London: HMSO.

DEPARTMENT OF PRICES AND CONSUMER PROTECTION (1978) *The Home Accident Surveillance System – Presentation of Twelve Months Data*, London: HMSO.

DEPARTMENT OF TRANSPORT (1979) *National Travel Survey: 1975/76 Report*, London: HMSO.

DOBASH, R. & DOBASH, R. (1982) 'The violent event' in Whitelegg, E., Arnot, M. et al. (eds.) *The Changing Experience of Women*, Oxford: Martin Robertson in association with The Open University.

DOOLEY, D. & CATALANO, R. (1980) 'Economic change as a cause of behavioural disorder', *Psychological Bulletin*, 87, 3: 450-68.

DOUGLAS, J. & BLOOMFIELD, J. (1958) *Children Under Five: The Results of a National Survey*, London: Allen & Unwin.

DOYAL, L. (1983) 'Women's health and the sexual division of labour', *Critical Social Policy*, 7, Summer: 21-33.

EARTHROWL, B. & STACEY, M. (1977) 'Social class and children in hospital' *Social Science and Medicine*, 11, 2: 83-8.

ELBOURNE, D. (1981) *Is the Baby All Right? Current Trends in Perinatal Health*, London: Junction Books.

ELECTRICITY COUNCIL (1979) *Electricity Users Survey – Summary Report*, prepared for the Electricity Council by MAS Survey Research Limited.

EPPRIGHT, E., FOX, H., FRYER, B., LAMKIN, G. & VIVIAN, N. (1969) 'Eating Behaviour of Preschool Children', *Journal of Nutrition Education*, 1: 16-19.

EQUAL OPPORTUNITIES COMMISSION (1982) *Caring for the Elderly and Handicapped: Community Care Policies and Women's Lives*, Manchester, EOC.

EQUAL OPPORTUNITIES COMMISSION (1983) *Seventh Annual Report: 1982*, Manchester: EOC.

ESSEN, J., FOGELMAN, K. & HEAD, J. (1978: a) 'Childhood housing experiences and school attainment', *Child: Care, Health & Development*, 4, 41-58.

ESSEN, J., FOGELMAN, K. & HEAD, J. (1978: b) 'Children's housing and their health and physical development', *Child: Care, Health and Development*, 4: 357-69.

EVASON, E. (1980: a) *Just Me and the Kids: A Study of Single Parent Families in Northern Ireland*, Belfast: EOC.

EVASON, E. (1980:b) *Ends That Won't Meet*, Poverty Research Series 8, London: Child Poverty Action Group.

EXTON-SMITH, A. (1980) 'Eating habits of the elderly' in Turner, M. (ed.) *Nutrition and Lifestyles*, London: Applied Science Publishers.

FAMILY SERVICE UNITS (1983) *Homes Fit for People*, London: FSU.

FERRI, E. (1976) *Growing Up in a One-Parent Family*, London: National Foundation for Educational Research in England and Wales.

FLORA PROJECT FOR HEART DISEASE PREVENTION (undated) *Coronary Disease: How to Protect Your Family*, London: The Flora Project.

FORREST, R. & MURIE, A. (1983) 'Residualisation and council housing: aspects of the changing social relations of housing tenure', *Journal of Social Policy*, 12, 4: 453-68

FREIDSON, E. (1961) *Patients' Views of Medical Practice*, New York: Russell Sage Foundation.

FRIIS, H., LAURITSEN, L. & STEEN, S. (1982) *One Parent Families and Poverty in the EEC*, Report to the Commission of European Communities, Copenhagen, December 1982.

GAVRON, H. (1966) *The Captive Wife*, Harmondsworth, Middlesex: Penguin.

GEORGE, V. & WILDING, P. (1972) *Motherless Families*, London: Routledge & Kegan Paul.

GOODWIN, B. (1982) 'The role of the bus' in Bus and Coach Council, *The Future of the Bus*, London: Bus and Coach Council.

GRAHAM, H. (1976) 'Smoking in pregnancy: the attitudes of expectant mothers', *Social Science & Medicine*, 10: 399-405.

GRAHAM, H. (1977) 'Women's attitudes to conception and pregnancy' in Chester, R. & Peel, J. (eds.) *Equalities and Inequalities in Family Life*, London: Academic Press.

GRAHAM, H. (1979: a) '"Prevention and Health: every mother's business": a comment on child health policy in the seventies' in Harris, C. (ed.) *The Sociology of the Family: New Directions for Britain*, University of Keele: Sociological Review Monograph 28.

GRAHAM, H. (1979: b) 'Problems in Antenatal Care', University of York: Department of Sociology.

GRAHAM, H. (1980: a) 'Family influences in early years on the eating habits of children' in Turner, M. (ed.) *Nutrition and Lifestyles*, London: Applied Science Publishers.

GRAHAM, H. (1980: b) 'Mothers' accounts of anger and aggression towards their babies' in Frude, N. (ed.) *Psychological Approaches to Child Abuse*, London: Batsford.

GRAHAM, H. (1982: a) 'Perceptions of Parenthood', *Health Education Journal*, 41, 4: 119-22.

GRAHAM, H. (1982: b) 'Coping or how mothers are seen and not heard' in Friedman, S. and Sarah, E. (eds.) *On the Problem of Men*, London: Women's Press.

GRAHAM, H. (1983: a) 'Health Education' in McPherson, A. and Anderson, A. (eds.) *Women's Problems in General Practice*, Oxford: Oxford University Press.

GRAHAM, H. (1983: b) 'Caring: A Labour of Love' in Finch, J. and Groves, D. (eds.) *A Labour of Love: Women, Work and Caring*, London: Routledge & Kegan Paul.

GRAHAM, H. (forthcoming) 'Providers, negotiators and mediators: Women as the hidden carers' in Olesen, V. and Lewin, E. *Women, Health and Policy*, New York: Tavistock.

GRAHAM, H. & McKEE, L. (1980) *The First Months of Motherhood*, Research Monograph No. 3, London: Health Education Council.

GRAY, A. (1979) 'The working class family as an economic unit' in Harris, C. (ed.) *The Sociology of the Family: New Directions for Britain*, University of Keele: Sociological Review Monograph 28.

GRIFFITH, A. (1982) 'Single parent families and education ideology: the reproduction of inequality' paper presented at the British Sociological Association Conference, *Gender and Society*, Manchester University.

HAKIM, C. (1982) 'The social consequences of high employment', *Journal of Social Policy*, 11, 4: 433-67.

HAMILL, L. (1978) *Wives as Sole and Joint Bread Winners*, Government Economic Service Working Papers, No. 13, London: HMSO.

HART, N. (1976) *When Marriage Ends*, London: Tavistock.

HASKEY, J. (1983) 'Children of divorcing couples', *Population Trends*, 31, Spring: 20-6.

HILLMAN, M., HENDERSON, I. & WHALLEY, A. (1974) *Mobility and Accessibility in the Outer Metropolitan Area*, Report to the Department of Environment, London: Political and Economic Planning.

HIPGRAVE, T. (1982) 'Lone fatherhood: a problematic status' in McKee, L. & O'Brien, M. (eds.) *The Father Figure*, London: Tavistock.

HOUSE OF COMMONS (1980) *Perinatal and Neonatal Mortality*, Second Report from the Social Services Committee, House of Commons Paper 663-1 (Session 1979-80), London: HMSO.

HOUSE OF COMMONS (1981) *Hansard*, 9 April, Vol. 2, No. 85, London: HMSO.

HOWE, P. & SCHILLER, M. (1952) 'Growth responses of the school child to changes in diet and environmental factors', *Journal of Applied Physiology*, 5: 51-5.

HUGHES, M., MAYALL, B., MOSS, P., PERRY, J., PETRIE, P. & PINKERTON, G. (1980) *Nurseries Now*, Harmondsworth, Middlesex: Penguin.

HUNT, A. (1968) *A Survey of Women's Employment*, London: OPCS.

HUNT, A., FOX, J. & MORGAN, M. (1973) *Families and Their Needs*, London: HMSO.

HUTTON, S. (1983) 'Housing Benefits and fuel', *Roof*, 8, 2: 7.

HUWS, U. (1982) *Your Job in the Eighties*, London: Pluto Press.

ILLSLEY, R. (1955) 'Social class selection and class differences in relation to stillbirth', *British Medical Journal*, 2: 1520-4.

INNER CITIES DIRECTORATE (1983) *1981 Census Information Note No. 2: Urban Deprivation*, London: Department of Environment, HMSO.

ITZIN, C. (1980) *Splitting Up: Single Parent Liberation*, London: Virago.

JACKSON, B. (1982) 'Single parent families' in Rapoport, R.N., Fogarty, M. & Rapoport, R. (eds.) *Families in Britain*, London: Routledge & Kegan Paul.

JACKSON, B. & JACKSON, S. (1979) *Child Minder*, London: Routledge & Kegan Paul.

JACOBSON, B. (1981) *The Lady Killers: Why Smoking is a Feminist Issue*, London: Pluto Press.

KELVIN, P. (1981) 'Work as a source of identity: the implications of unemployment', *British Journal of Guidance and Counselling*, 9, 1: 2-11.

KERR, M. & CHARLES, N. (1982) 'Food as an indicator of social relations', paper presented to the Annual Conference of the British Sociological Association, *Gender and Society*, University of Manchester.

KERR, M. & CHARLES, N. (1983) *Attitudes to the Feeding and Nutrition of Young Children: Preliminary Report*, University of York.

KINCAID, J. (1973) *Poverty and Inequality in Britain*, Harmondsworth, Middlesex: Penguin.

KLEIN, V. (1974) *Women in Employment*, Paris: Organisation for Economic Co-operation and Development.

KOOS, E. (1954) *The Health of Regionville: What the People Felt & Did About It*, Columbia: Columbia University Press.

LAND, H. (1977) 'Inequalities in large families: more of the same or or different?' in Chester, R. & Peel, J. (eds.) *Equalities and Inequalities in Family Life*, London: Academic Press.

LAND, H. (1981) *Parity begins at home*, EOC/SSRC Joint Panel on Equal Opportunities, Manhcester: EOC/SSRC.

LAND, H. (1983) 'Poverty and gender: the distribution of resources within the family' in Brown, M. (ed.) *The Structure of Disadvantage*, London: Heinemann.

LANG, T. (1983) 'Food and welfare', *Bulletin on Social Policy*, 13, Spring: 13-19.

LAWRENCE, M. (1979) 'Anorexia nervosa — the control paradox', *Women's Studies International Quarterly*, 2:93-101.

LAYARD, R., PIACHAUD, D., STEWART, M. (1978) *The Causes of Poverty*, Royal Commission on the Distribution of Income and Wealth, Background Paper to Report No. 6, London: HMSO.

LE GRAND, J. (1982) *The Strategy of Inequality*, London: Allen & Unwin.

LETTS, P. (1983) *Double Struggle: Sex Discrimination and One Parent Families*, London: National Council for One Parent Families.

LISTER, R. & EMETT, T. (1976) *Under the Safety Net*, Poverty Pamphlet 25, London: Child Poverty Action Group.

LITMAN, T. (1974) 'The family as a basic unit in health and medical care', *Social Science and Medicine*, 8:495-519.

LITTLEWOOD, J. & TINKER, A. (1981) *Families in Flats*, Department of Environment, London: HMSO.

LORANT, J. (1981) *Poor and Powerless: Fuel problems and Disconnections*, Poverty Pamphlet 52, London: Child Poverty Action Group.

LOW PAY REVIEW (1983) 'Research & statistics', *Low Pay Review*, 13, May: 23-4

MACFARLANE, A. & ARMSTRONG, B. (1983) 'Cuts in the government statistical service', *Radical Statistics*, 27: 8-10.

MACFARLANE, A. & FOX, J. (1978) 'Child deaths from accident and violence', *Population Trends*, 12, Spring: 22-7.

MACFARLANE, A. & MUGFORD, M. (1984) *Birth Counts*, London: HMSO.

MACINTYRE, S. (1977) *Single and Pregnant*, London: Croom Helm.

MACLEAN, M. & EEKELAAR, J. (1983) *Children and Divorce: Economic Factors*, Wolfson College, Oxford: Centre for Socio-Legal Studies.

McCLELLAND, J. (1982) *A Little Pride and Dignity: The Importance of Child Benefit*, Poverty Pamphlet 54, London: Child Poverty Action Group.

McKEE, L. (1983) 'Wives and the recession' paper presented to the Central Birmingham Health Education Department conference on *Unemployment and its Effect upon the Family*, Birmingham.

McKEE, L. & O'BRIEN, M. (1982) *The Father Figure*, London: Tavistock.

McKEOWN, T. (1979) *The Role of Medicine*, Oxford: Basil Blackwell.

McKINLAY, J. (1973) 'Social networks, lay consultation and help-seeking behaviour', *Social Forces*, 5: 275-92.

McNAY, M. & POND, C. (1980) *Low Pay and Family Poverty*, Study Commission on the Family, occasional paper No. 2, London: Study Commission on the Family.

MADGE, N. (ed.) (1983) *Families at Risk*, London: Heinemann

MARSDEN, D. (1973) *Mothers Alone: Poverty and the Fatherless Family*, Harmondsworth, Middlesex: Penguin.

MARSDEN, D. & DUFF, E. (1975) *Workless*, Harmondsworth, Middlesex: Penguin.

MECHANIC, D. (1964) 'The influence of mothers on their children's health attitudes and behaviour', *Pediatrics* 33: 444-53.

MILLAR, J. (1983) *Family Men*, DHSS Cohort Study of Unemployed Men, No. 4, London: DHSS

MINISTRY OF AGRICULTURE, FISHERIES AND FOOD (1982) *Household Food Consumption and Expenditure 1980*, London: HMSO.

MOSS, P. (1980) 'Parents at work' in Moss, P. & Fonda, N. (eds.) *Work and the Family*, London: Temple Smith.

MOSS, P. & LEWIS, I. (1977) 'Mental stress in mothers of pre-school children in inner-London', *Psychological Medicine*, 7: 641-52.

MURCOTT, A. (1982: a) '"It's a pleasure to cook for him": food, mealtimes and gender in some South Wales households' in Gamarnikow, E., Morgan, D., Purvis, J. & Taylorshot, D. (eds.) *The Public and the Private*, London: Heinemann.

MURCOTT, A. (1982: b) 'On the social significance of the "cooked dinner" in South Wales', *Social Science Information*, 21, 4-5: 677-95.

MURCOTT, A. (1983) 'Cooking and the cooked' in Murcott, A. (ed.) *The Sociology of Food and Eating*, Aldershot, Hants.: Gower.

MURIE, A. (1983) *Housing Inequality and Deprivation*, London: Heinemann.

NANDY, L. (1982) 'Families and unemployment: a report from the north west', University of Bradford: School of Applied Social Studies.

NATIONAL CONSUMER COUNCIL (1983) *Cracking Up: Building Faults in Council Homes*, London: NCC.

NATIONAL COUNCIL FOR ONE PARENT FAMILIES (1980) *One Parent Families 1980* London: NCOPF.

NATIONAL COUNCIL FOR ONE PARENT FAMILIES (1982) *One Parent Families 1982*, London: NCOPF.

NATIONAL COUNCIL FOR ONE PARENT FAMILIES (1983) *One Parent Families 1983*, London: NCOPF.

NEWSOM, J. & NEWSOM, E. (1970) *Four Years Old in an Urban Community*, Harmondsworth, Middlesex: Penguin.

NICHOLLS, T. (1979) 'Social class: official, sociological and Marxist' in Irvine, J., Miles, I. and Evans, J. (eds.) *Demystifying Social Statistics*, London: Pluto Press.

NIELSEN, J. & ENDO, R. (1983) 'Marital status and socio-economic status: the case of female-headed families', *International Journal of Women's Studies*, 6, 2: 130-47.

NISSEL, M. (1980) 'Women in government statistics: basic concepts and assumptions', *EOC Research Bulletin*, 4, Autumn: 5-28.

NISSEL, M. & BONNERJEA, L. (1983) *Family care for the handicapped elderly: who pays?* London: Policy Studies Institute.

NIXON, J. (1979) *Fatherless Families on Family Income Supplement*, Research Report 4, DHSS, London: HMSO.

OAKLEY, A. (1974) *The Sociology of Housework*, Oxford: Martin Robertson.

O'BRIEN, M. (1982) 'Becoming a lone father: differential patterns and experiences' in McKee, L. and O'Brien, M. (eds.) *The Father Figure*, London: Tavistock.

OFFICE OF POPULATION CENSUSES AND SURVEYS (1980) *General Household Survey 1978*, London: HMSO.

OFFICE OF POPULATION CENSUSES AND SURVEYS (1982: a) *General Household Survey 1980*, London: HMSO.

OFFICE OF POPULATION CENSUSES AND SURVEYS (1982: b) *County Reports*, CEN 81, London: HMSO.

OFFICE OF POPULATION CENSUSES AND SURVEYS (1982: c)

Mortality Statistics 1978, 1979: Perinatal & infant (social and biological factors) Series DH3 No 7, London: HMSO.

OLIVER, J. (1983) 'The caring wife' in Finch, J. & Groves, D. (eds.) *A Labour of Love: Women, Work and Caring*, London: Routledge & Kegan Paul.

OREN, L. (1974) 'The welfare of women in labouring families: England, 1860-1950', in Hartman, M. & Banner, L. (eds.) *Clio's Consciousness Raised: New Perspectives on the History of Women*, London: Harper & Row.

OSBORN, A. & MORRIS, T. (1979) 'The rationale for a composite index of social class and its evaluation', *British Journal of Sociology*, 30, 1:39-60.

PAHL, J. (1980) 'Patterns of money management within marriage', *Journal of Social Policy*, 9, 3: 313-35.

PERKINS, E. (1980) 'The pattern of women's attendance at antenatal classes: is this good enough?' *Health Education Journal*, 39, 1:3-9.

PIACHAUD, D. (1979) *The Cost of a Child*, Poverty Pamphlet 43, London: Child Poverty Action Group.

PIACHAUD, D. (1981) *Children and Poverty*, Poverty Research Series 9, London: Child Poverty Action Group.

PIACHAUD, D. (1982) 'Patterns of income and expenditure within families', *Journal of Social Policy*, 11, 4:469-82.

PICKUP, L. (1981) *Housewives' Mobility and Travel Patterns*, LR971, Department of the Environment/Department of Transport, Crowthorne, Berkshire: Transport and Road Research Laboratory.

PILL, R. & STOTT, N. (1982) 'Concepts of illness causation and responsibility: some preliminary data from a sample of working class mothers', *Social Science and Medicine*, 16: 43-52.

POLITICS OF HEALTH GROUP (1980) *Food and Profit*, London: POHG.

POLLERT, A. (1981) *Girls, Wives, Factory Lives*, London: Macmillan.

POND, C. & POPAY, J. (1983) 'Tackling inequalities at their source' in Glennerster, H. (ed.) *The Future of the Welfare State*, London: Heinemann.

POPAY, J., RIMMER, L. & ROSSITER, C. (1983) *One Parent Families: Parents, Children and Public Policy*, Study Commission on the Family, occasional paper No. 12, London: Study Commission on the Family.

POTTER, J. (1982) *Public Transport*, London: National Consumer Council.

RAMSDEN, S. & SMEE, C. (1981) 'The health of unemployed men: DHSS cohort study', *Employment Gazette*, 89, 9:397-401.

RAPOPORT, R. N., FOGARTY, M. & RAPOPORT, R. (eds.)(1982)

Families in Britain, British Family Responsibility Committee, Institute of Family and Environmental Research, London: Routledge & Kegan Paul.

REDFERN, P. (1982) 'Profile of our cities', *Population Trends*, 30, Autumn: 21-32.

REPORT OF THE COMMITTEE ON CHILD HEALTH SERVICES (1976) 'Fit for the Future', Cmnd 6684, Vol. I (the Court Report) London: HMSO.

REPORT OF THE COMMITTEE ON ONE PARENT FAMILIES (1974), Cmnd 5629, Vol. 1 (the Finer Report) London: HMSO.

REPORT OF THE ROYAL COMMISSION ON THE NATIONAL HEALTH SERVICE (1979), Cmnd 7615, (Chairman: Sir Alec Merrison), London: HMSO.

REVIEW BODY (1981) 'Coronary prone behaviour and coronary heart disease: a critical review', *Circulation*, 63: 1199-215.

RICHARDS, M. & DYSON, M. (1982) *Separation, Divorce and the Development of Children: A Review*, University of Cambridge: Child Care and Development Group.

RICHARDSON, P. (1977) 'York Branch study of fuel debts', *Poverty*, 36: 16-17.

RICHMAN, N. (1974) 'The effects of housing on pre-school children and their mothers', *Developmental Medicine and Child Neurology*, 16: 53-8.

RICHMAN, N. (1976) 'Depression in mothers of young children', *Journal of Child Psychology and Psychiatry*, 17: 75-8.

RICHMAN, N., STEVENSON, J., & GRAHAM, P. (1982) *Preschool to School: A Behavioural Study*, London: Academic Press.

RIMMER, L. & POPAY, J. (1982) *Employment Trends and the Family*, London: Study Commission on the Family.

ROLL, J. (1983) 'Facts and figures', *Poverty*, 55: 10-14.

ROTTER, J. (1954) *Social Learning and Clinical Psychology*, Eaglewood Cliffs, New Jersey: Prentice Hall.

ROWBOTHAM, S. (1973) *Woman's Consciousness, Man's World*, Harmondsworth, Middlesex: Penguin.

ROWNTREE, B.S. (1941) *Poverty and Progress*, London: Longman.

ROYAL COLLEGE OF GENERAL PRACTITIONERS (1982) *Healthier Children — Thinking Prevention*, Report from General Practice 22, London: RCGP.

ROYAL COLLEGE OF PHYSICIANS OF LONDON (1977) *Smoking or Health* (Third Report), London: Pitman.

SCHWENK, T. & HUGHES, C. (1983) 'The family as patient in family medicine: rhetoric or reality?' *Social Science and Medicine*, 17: 1-16.

SHIMMIN, S., McNALLY, J. & LIFF, S. (1981) 'Pressures on women engaged in factory work', *Employment Gazette*, 89, 8: 344-9.

SIMPSON, R. (1980) *For the Sake of the Children*, London: National Council for One Parent Families.

SKEGG, D., DOLL, R. & PERRY, J. (1977) 'Use of medicine in general practice', *British Medical Journal*, 1,6076: 1561-3.

SMITH, B. (1983) 'Prices and the poor', *Low Pay Review*, 9: 1-6.

SMITH, D. & DAVID, S. (1974) *Women Look at Psychiatry*, New York: Press Gang Publishers.

SMITH, I. (1981) 'Cause of death: attitudes of mind', *Times Health Supplement*, 7: 12-13.

SMITHELLS, R., SHEPPARD, S. et al. (1980) 'Possible prevention of neural-tube defects, by periconceptual vitamin supplementation', *Lancet*, I: 339-40.

SPENCE, J., WALTON, W., MILLER, F., COURT, S. (1954) *A Thousand Families in Newcastle-upon-Tyne: An Approach to the Study of Health and Illness in Children*, Oxford: Oxford University Press.

SPENCER, N. (1979) 'An education for health educators?' in Anderson, D., Perkins, E. & Spencer, N. *Who Knows Best in Health Education?* Occasional paper No. 19, University of Nottingham, Leverhulme Health Education Project.

SPENCER, N. (1980) *Parent Identification and Management of Illness in Infants*, Unpublished M. Phil. thesis, University of Nottingham.

SPENCER, N. (forthcoming) 'Mother's recognition of the ill child' in Macfarlane, J. (ed.) *Progress in Child Health*, London: Churchill Livingstone/Longman.

SPRING RICE, M. (1939) *Working class wives: their health and conditions*, Penguin (republished 1981, London: Virago).

STELLMAN, J. (1977) *Women's Work, Women's Health*, New York: Pantheon Books.

STERN, J. (1983) 'Social mobility and the interpretation of social class mortality differentials', *Journal of Social Policy*, 12: 27-49.

STRONG, P. (1979) *The Ceremonial Order of the Clinic: Patients, Doctors and Medical Bureaucracies*, London: Routledge & Kegan Paul.

SUPPLEMENTARY BENEFITS COMMISSION (1979) *Annual Report 1978*, London: HMSO.

SUTHERLAND, I. (ed.) (1979) *Health Education: Perspectives and Choices*, London: Allen & Unwin.

TAX, M. (1970) *Woman and Her Mind, The Story of Daily Life*, Cambridge, Mass.: Bread and Roses.

THOMAS, G. & SHANNON, C. (1982) 'Technology and household labour: are the times a-changing?' Paper presented at the British Sociological Association Annual Conference, *Gender and Society*, University of Manchester.

TINKER, A. (1981) *The Elderly in Modern Society*, London: Longman.

TODD, J. & JONES, L. (1972) *Matrimonial Property*, Social Survey Division, London: HMSO.

TODD, J. & WALKER, A. (1980) *People as Pedestrians*, Social Survey Division, London: HMSO.

TONES, K. (1977) *Effectiveness and Efficiency in Health Education*, Scottish Health Education Unit.

TOWNSEND, P. (1979) *Poverty in the United Kingdom*, Harmondsworth, Middlesex: Penguin.

TOWNSEND, P. (1981) 'Towards equality in health through social policy', *International Journal of Health Services*, 11, 1:63-75.

TOWNSEND, P. & DAVIDSON, N. (1982) *Inequalities in Health*, Harmondsworth, Middlesex: Penguin.

TUCKETT, D. (1979) 'Choices for health education: a sociological view' in Sutherland, I. (ed.) *Health Education: Perspectives and Choices*, London: Allen & Unwin.

TUDOR HART, J. (1971) 'The inverse care law', *Lancet*, 1: 405-12.

UNITED STATES COMMISSION ON CIVIL RIGHTS (1974) *Women and Poverty*, Staff Report, Washington, DC: US Government Printing Office.

VOYSEY, M. (1975) *A Constant Burden: the Reconstitution of Family Life*, London: Routledge & Kegan Paul.

WADSWORTH, J., BURNELL, I., TAYLOR, B. & BUTLER, N. (1983) 'Family type and accidents in pre-school children', *Journal of Epidemiology and Community Health*, 37, 2: 100-4.

WALKER, A. (1983) 'Care for elderly people: a conflict between women and the state' in Finch, J. & Groves, D. (eds.) *A Labour of Love: Women, Work and Caring*, London: Routledge & Kegan Paul.

WALLERSTEIN, J. & BERLIN KELLY, J. (1980) *Surviving the Break-up: How Children Cope With Divorce*, London: Grant McIntyre.

WEISS, R. (1979) *Going it alone: the family life and social situation of the single parent*, New York: Basic Books.

WEISSMAN, M. & KLERMAN, G. (1977) 'Symptom patterns in primary and secondary depression: a comparison', *Archives of General Psychiatry*, 34:854-62.

WILKIN, D. (1979) *Caring for the Mentally Handicapped Child*, London: Croom Helm.

WILSON, H. & HERBERT, G. (1978) *Parents and Their Children in the Inner City*, London: Routledge & Kegan Paul.

WINFIELD, M. (1983) *The Human Cost of Fuel Disconnection*, London: Family Service Units.

204 *Women, Health and the Family*

WOMAN'S OWN (1975) 'Housekeeping survey', *Woman's Own*, 20 September.

WOMEN'S CO-OPERATIVE GUILD (1915) *Maternity: Letters from Working Women*, Bell & Sons (republished 1978, London: Virago).

WORKING GROUP ON HEALTH INEQUALITIES (1980) *Inequalities in Health*, (the Black Report) London: DHSS.

WYNN, M. & WYNN, A. (1981) 'Historical associations of congenital malformations', *International Journal of Environmental Studies*, 17: 7-12.

ZOLA, I. (1973) 'Pathways to the doctor — from person to patient', *Social Science and Medicine*, 7:677-89.

Index